I0407753

BLACK WOMBMAN

A Novel
by Amirah Bellamy

Black Wombman.   Copyright © 2015 by Amirah Bellamy. All Rights Reserved. Printed in the United States of America.   No part of this book may be used or reproduced in any manner whatsoever without written permission except in the case of brief quotations embodied in critical articles or reviews.

For information contact
twenty6dimension@gmail.com

BLACK WOMBMAN

is dedicated to all the Carbos across the planet. May you all continue to awaken from your slumber and follow the call to illuminate from within….. It's our time!!!

ACKNOWLEDGMENTS

I thank my Higher Self for an ever evolving awareness of my true desires as they continue to awaken and enlighten me revealing to me the power within and the manifestation of a most wonderful life, satisfaction and happiness. I thank the will of my spirit within for being open to receive and focused on my higher purpose in the face of life's contrast and idle concerns of mundane matters….

1

Goddess. Cyno. Spako. **Lupae. The Great Bitch.** Bitch! Stop bitching. Son of a bitch. Bitch ass nigga! Bitch please. No that bitch didn't. Bitch better have my money. Bitches ain't shit. Ain't that about a bitch! Life's a bitch. Karma's a bitch. So long bitches. Why are you acting like a bitch? Queen bitch. Sometimes I can be a real bitch. Wutup bitches? Fuck that bitch! Fat bitch. Dudes with money get all the bitches. Dumb bitch. You's a nasty bitch. Bitches and hoes. Stank bitches. Where my bitches at?

****

……….. **Nigga** anxiously returned to Bast smiling ear to ear with a smile that was brighter than sunshine. The moment she saw him she ran up to him and gave him a hug that was bigger than the universe.

"So are you ready to party now my love?" Bast asked smiling.

"Do you have to ask? And I hope ya'll got all the trimmings for a *real* party, the way *we* do it, cause this party needs to last for at least a few million years! So break out the bubbly, the forties, the pints, the j's, the grill, the cards, the dominoes, the horseshoes and the shit-talking. Then prepare *our* room with all of my favorite outfits with the blessing that is your ass out because I don't know how long *we're* gonna be *partying*!" Nigga said excitedly.

"Wow you're funny! You are *really* funny! And you know what? I already did all of that! Stop acting like you know me God," Bast said smiling

"Oh I'm not acting. You know who I am. Now get over here and *show* me that you know who I am!" Nigga ordered.......

Following the revolution all was well for the next several years. Though as time went on Bast and the others began to realize that the next degree of cleansing had yet to take place and soon enough it did.

The first signs of that began as subtle changes. For Bast, one in particular was that her feelings for Nigga began to take a bit of an unexpected shift. She noticed it one night while laying in the bed awake as she nestled on Nigga's chest.

Deep in thought Bast reminisced on what was to come. More importantly she was struck with an onslaught of haunting images from her past, a very distant past and she wasn't the only one.

Several other Queens were also suddenly developing the ability to recall past lives, each experiencing it in a unique way. Yet, each of them recalled a shared past that was shocking and appalling, the memories of which were torturous. However, it was exactly what they needed to break free from the prison that they had for so long been deluded by.

Meanwhile, it seemed that a distance was growing between the Gods and their Queens. Yet it wasn't so much distance as it was an emotional shift. Bast wasn't the only one that noticed it. Like the recalling of past lives, many other queens had expressed similar observations. In fact, there was one report of it that was most intriguing and somewhat troubling and it involved Bast's twin sister, Aset....

(TO BE CONTINUED)

2

Aset looked around at everyone sharing the same train car as she with an expression of utter disgust. Aset preferred to take the train to work rather than drive to avoid sitting in traffic. That day she couldn't quite pinpoint why, but she was just in one of her funks. She'd been in one for the past couple of days.

Something was bugging her, but what it was hadn't yet revealed itself. This happened to Aset frequently. It usually occurred when something was off and usually that something was her man, Siris, whom she called Si for short.

They'd been together for two years and were just about to celebrate their 3rd anniversary. Aset couldn't believe they'd actually made it that far. She'd been through more ups and downs with him than she'd ever been through in the thirty plus years she'd been alive.

As she rode on the train she thought to herself that she hoped that she wasn't about to experience another of their downs because she'd had it with him. Though the ups with him were really good, the downs were pretty bad. Lately she'd gotten to the point where she just didn't think she could take another down with him.

As she dove deeper into her musings Aset thought to herself that Siris was no God. He was just a vile pestilence infecting everyone he came into contact with the disease of his existence. He was just another brother with an over-inflated ego trying to make something significant of his pathetic, worthless self, which somehow included blaming everything undesirable on the women in his life.

She was always to blame and as she listened to the hum of the train that had somehow put her in a trance-like state Aset thought to herself that she was over it. She was so much more than the blame of all the things *wrong* in Si's pathetic life and in her heightened state of prophetic insight she saw the day was soon coming that it was about to be more than evident. She simply had to cut through the bull-shit long enough to remember.

Siris was two years older than Aset, but she always felt that she was a lot more mature than he was. Siris was a rather handsome guy standing about 6 feet, 4 inches tall with a medium, semi-muscular build. He was medium brown complexioned, wore his hair in a short, curly afro faded around the edges and had the most intense, gorgeous eyes. Aset would always notice women staring at him and though Siris never disrespected her by returning the glance something told her that he probably enjoyed the attention when she wasn't around.

Aset was just as good a looker. Her looks too solicited quite a bit of attention from the opposite sex. Aset was about 5 feet, 4 inches at around 130 pounds. She was just a half shade lighter than Siris and wore her hair in a huge natural, blow out, which hung about halfway down her back. Her most stunning feature was her body. She had an hourglass figure that was the envy of most women who ever laid eyes on her. Yet, while the women were envious the men were entranced by Aset as her physique alone made her quite the master at the art of seduction.

Together Siris and Aset were pure magnetism. It seemed that when they walked into a room together all eyes were instantly magnetically drawn to them. For that reason the women were jealous of Aset and the men were envious of Siris.

Ironically enough Aset and Siris met one day on the train as they were both headed home from work. Siris worked in downtown

D.C. as an architectural draftsman for a mid-sized architectural firm at the time, while Aset was working in Vienna, Virginia as a HR consultant for a small software company.

Siris boarded the train and sat in the seat adjacent to Aset who had already been on the train for some time. As the train made it's way through several downtown stops before entering the suburbs of Maryland the train gradually began to empty.

Meanwhile, from the moment that Siris had boarded the train his eyes were instantly drawn to and stayed glued to Aset. When his eyes landed on her he thought that she was absolutely stunning and wanted desperately to get the opportunity to meet her. So as the person who was sharing the seat with Aset got off the train and Aset moved over to the inside seat Siris saw his opportunity and immediately seized it swiftly moving to occupy the vacant seat.

"I hope you don't mind my sitting here," Siris said gazing into Aset's mesmerizing eyes for confirmation.

"Oh no, not at all. I was wondering when you would make your way over here," Aset said smiling.

"Oh yeah, sorry about that. I didn't mean to stare, but all the same I'm sure you get that all the time," Siris replied.

"Hmmm not exactly. You weren't even *trying* to be discreet, Aset laughed.

"Oh so you got jokes," Siris said.

"I try," Aset answered.

"That's ok. You're right. I *was* checking you out. I figured there was no need in hiding my interest. Besides that when I saw you I figured there was no way I was going to let you get away. You are gorgeous!" Siris said gawking.

"Well that's rather presumptuous of you. How do you know I *haven't* gotten away?" Aset asked.

"Because I know destiny when I see it. Right now I see it as you and me so here we are," Siris said with a light chuckle.

"Well, I *love* your confidence. After all confidence is key," Aset said playing hard to get.

She did enjoy the chase a bit, probably a lot more than most. For her the best part of the chase was that in the end *she* got to choose and she *always* made sure that she had a nice selection to choose from.

Siris was correct. Aset *did* get hit on a lot. It was a daily occurrence. Some days she was in the mood to entertain it and other days she wasn't. Lucky for Siris he caught her on a good day when she happened to be in the mood to be entertained.

Even better, Aset was also in the mood for a bit of risk-taking so she decided to make things even more difficult for Siris. She knew that he would soon ask her for a way to keep in touch and she decided that she would not make it that easy for him. Instead, she chose to let destiny decide.

So as her stop approached Aset began to gather her things. Then, just as expected Siris asked for her phone number.

Getting up to exit the train Aset said, "Hmmm, well like you I too know destiny when I see it so I'm going to let destiny decide if you get my phone number."

Then with that Aset abruptly exited the train leaving Siris looking heart-broken. As the train pulled off and he watched Aset walking in the opposite direction down the platform he felt a devastation that penetrated the pit of his stomach. No woman had ever before done such a thing to him.

For a moment he felt a pang of anger. Then a thought crossed his mind that perhaps Aset was right. If it was meant to be then he would see her again. Though as much as he tried to remain optimistic it didn't last beyond another couple of days because he did not see Aset again.

As the days passed his anger returned. He just could not seem to get her off of his mind. He was also angry at himself because he'd forgotten to even ask for her name.

Then when he thought about it he realized that he didn't really know *anything* about her. He was even more upset with himself for not using his time more wisely to get more information about her. Had he gotten her name he could have at least been able to perhaps look her up.

On top of that thousands of people rode on the train everyday which made the odds of seeing her again slim to none. As it was, that was the first time he'd ever seen her. Besides that who knew if they'd ever be on the same train car again. He didn't even know what stop she boarded the train on.

Siris was distraught over the thought of it and he tried with all of his will to stop thinking about her. Yet no matter what he did to try to distract himself he failed miserably every time. Another day had come and gone and Siris still hadn't seen Aset.

Meanwhile, Aset was also still thinking of Siris, which was odd for her. With so many guys hitting on her daily, rarely did she continue thinking about them. Yet there was something a little different about Siris that had intrigued her. It wasn't his looks because plenty of fine brothahs approached her. It wasn't really his pick-up line either because nothing about it was the least bit original. She wondered to herself what it was, but came up empty. So after a few days had passed Aset too began to hope that she would see Siris again.

It wasn't until about three weeks later that the two of them finally crossed paths again. Yet as destiny would have it, it wasn't even on the train.

3

It was a Saturday afternoon and Aset was enjoying one of her favorite pastimes. Aside from drawing and painting Aset loved going to the bookstore. Though it was old-fashioned to read hard copies of books while most read electronic versions there was something about the hard copy of books that Aset enjoyed. Perhaps it was that doing so stimulated all of her senses or perhaps it was more engaging to be out and about with other people that gave her a sense of interconnectedness. Whatever, it was Aset absolutely loved it and so her visits to the bookstore occurred quite often.

One day Aset was in the parking lot of Bowie Town Center, which was located in the suburbs of Prince George's County Maryland. When she parked her car and got out who did she happen to see, but Siris who was actually leaving as he headed to his car which was parked about two cars down from Aset's.

"I can't believe it!" Siris said with a huge grin plastered across his face.

"Oh is that so. I thought you knew destiny when you saw it," Aset laughed.

"Ha ha, funny, funny," Siris said, "I do, but I never expected to run into you here. Where are you headed? Would you like some company?" he said looking around as if to make sure Aset was there alone.

"Actually, as destiny would have it, I wouldn't mind that at all and yes I'm here alone. I'm just heading to the bookstore, a favorite pastime of mine" Aset replied smiling.

"Well that's perfect because as destiny would have it, now so am I. Shall we?" Siris said extending his arm outward in the direction of the bookstore.

Aset looked at Siris then at his arm, smiled and nodded as she walked ahead. The bookstore turned out to be a perfect first date for Aset and Siris because they learned that they shared many of the same interests. Also as destiny would have it they were both avid readers and specifically enjoyed reading about the esoteric.

As they talked they discovered that they had studied much of the same things over the years and what was even more ironic was that their studies both complimented one another's. While Aset studied the esoteric from a more spiritual perspective, Siris studied it from a more scientific one.

The more Aset got to know Siris, the more intrigued she became with him. He was definitely making his way to the top of her list of prospects. Though there still was another who was close on his heels so there was no telling in what direction the scales would ultimately tip.

The two must have stayed at the bookstore talking for hours. For both of them it was the best unplanned date ever. When it was time to part ways Siris asked Aset for her phone number. He wasn't sure if she was still going to play hard to get so he really didn't know what to expect.

Though, luckily she made things easier for him by giving him her number. He was confident that through more conversations he could win her over, which he eventually did. It took quite a bit of time though because she was still seeing the other prospect with whom Aset was just as intrigued.

In the end it was actually a very tough decision for Aset. In addition to the other prospect someone from her past had resurfaced around the same time that she started talking to Siris. It was an ex that she actually had regrets about leaving. His name was Jalil.

Jalil was a breathtakingly beautiful brothah, one of the most gorgeous creatures to ever walk the earth in Aset's opinion. In addition to that he treated Aset like a queen. He showered her with loving gestures every opportunity that he got.

Jalil and Aset dated for a little over 2 years and then Aset one day just broke up with him without giving any signs or warning that she was going to do so. She broke up with Jalil because she felt that their relationship wasn't as much a priority for him as it was for her. Jalil had quite a bit of unsettled things going on in his life at the time and Aset simply didn't want to wait any longer for him to resolve them.

Jalil had married at the young age of 20 and consequently had just recently divorced when he met Aset. It was that which led Aset to draw the conclusion about the future of their relationship that she did. She felt that he still wasn't over his ex-wife. She grew tired of hearing about her and having to witness his getting so emotional over the issues that they had. Jalil also tended to take things that his wife did out on Aset at times and that greatly disturbed her. She had expressed her dissatisfaction about it to Jalil several times, but it didn't seem to sink in.

Jalil's wife had been unfaithful to him, which was what led to their divorce. Then to add insult to injury she moved the guy that she was cheating with into the house that she shared with Jalil. Then one day when he came home from work to his surprise they were both there waiting for him accompanied by the police to put him out of his own house. It was ugly and the split was devastating to Jalil. It seemed he would never truly get over it. At least that's how Aset saw it, which was why she decided to break things off with him. She felt that after going through something so devastating he needed time to heal the emotional scars before moving on to the next relationship.

Besides that, what really finalized her decision was that she had begun to notice little changes in his behavior once the honeymoon phase of their relationship fizzled. All of sudden there were long periods of time that he wasn't accessible. He started 'hanging out with his 'friends' more, or so he said. He seemed a bit more argumentative and a lot more often. In fact, at times it was as if he was actually purposely *trying* to start arguments.

Aset knew all too well of that ploy. It usually meant that the brothah was either looking for an out or trying to find a reason to justify a disappearance for a day or two. Aset knew that what was really going on was that Jalil had started seeing other women.

She tried not to take it personally as she knew that in his mind it was the big get back for what his ex-wife had done. However, *she* was not his ex-wife and *she* had not during any time been unfaithful in their relationship. Thus, she didn't deserve to be dogged out for what the last woman did.

She couldn't figure out why time and time again she had to keep getting punished for what his ex-wife had done and so for Aset Jalil's unfaithfulness was the final straw! She was done being punished for what another woman had done to him. As far as she was concerned he needed to grow up and she wasn't about to waste anymore time waiting for him to do so!

So rather than allowing things to get any worse Aset decided that it was best they just part ways while they were still on good terms. Of course Jalil was heart-broken. He didn't understand why Aset broke up with him when in his mind all he did was love her. Sure he had other women, but Aset didn't know about any of them, or so he thought.

What he *didn't* know was that Aset was very different from most women. Not only was Aset highly intelligent, but she was very intuitive. She had the most uncanny ability to somehow *know* certain things. Whenever things were off she could just *feel* it. It mostly came out in her art.

Aset was a painter so she would paint whatever came to mind and more often than not what she painted revealed undeniable truths that even *she* sometimes couldn't believe. In fact, there was one that she had of Jalil that was more than she could take and it devastated her.

4

Aset's talents as a painter far surpassed her skills as an HR Consultant. Thus, unlike her dead end career as a HR Consultant Aset's professional painting career was quickly advancing. She actually had gotten her artwork into several art museums all over the country. At the time that she was dating Jalil her paintings were quickly gaining a bit of notoriety and so her artwork was being featured at quite a few events throughout the city.

There was one show in particular that Aset would never forget. It was her birthday weekend and she had a pretty big local show that Saturday night. She had prepared to unveil a special piece that she had made of Jalil and was anxious to show it to him at the event.   Though as the gig approached she heard less and less from Jalil.   In fact, she hadn't heard from him in over a week, which was quite unusual since they typically spoke several times a day.

Ironically enough about a couple of weeks prior Jalil had expressed to Aset that he felt he needed some space to resolve some issues and to emotionally get over his ex-wife. Aset agreed and so he and Aset weren't seeing one another as frequently.   In fact, she pulled back and decided not to call him at all to give him the freedom to call her when he was ready. Though as the days went by and Aset didn't hear from Jalil she knew that their relationship was done.   She could feel it in her spirit.

Nonetheless, she still had the gig and she had told Jalil about the event at least a month prior with a few reminders along the way.   Initially, he had told her that he would be there so she expected that he would honor his word and attend.

Needless to say Jalil did not attend the event and Aset was devastated.   She couldn't believe how unsupportive and insensitive he had been.

In her highly emotional state later that night Aset had an irresistible impulse to paint. So she got out of bed and began painting. Whenever she painted like that it was as if she was possessed. So she painted the images of what was transmitted to her from what seemed to be a higher force.

By the time she finished Aset looked on to see that the painting was of Jalil. Accompanying Jalil was a woman. She was an attractive dark complexioned sistah with long, beautiful locs. In the painting the two of them were spending the weekend together at some hotel. As Aset looked down at the finished piece it pierced her heart like a dagger. She knew with everything in her being that Jalil was at the hotel with the woman in the painting right then and it outraged her. In her anger Aset destroyed the painting covering it all with black paint.

After that incident Aset vowed to never allow herself to be hurt that way again.

Consequently, she broke things off with Jalil without ever even giving him an explanation as to why. In fact, she never spoke of it to anyone.

However, despite what Jalil had done Aset knew that it was his way of lashing back out at women for what his ex-wife had done to him. That was why she figured he needed time to heal from that relationship before moving on. Getting into a relationship before being emotionally ready caused Jalil to unduly lash out at Aset. Yet, Jalil never saw it that way.

So for months Jalil tried to get Aset to come back to him, but it was to no avail. Since she had never actually told him why she ended things with him he was plagued with unanswered questions. As far as he knew things at that time were in a good space with them. Even after the birthday weekend fiasco he had profusely apologized and thought that he had made his way back into her heart and that all was forgiven. Aset acted as though it was and so in his mind since then things had never been better between them. Yet, unbeknownst to him Aset was having great difficulty erasing the vision of Jalil and the other woman from her mind. It hurt her to the core.

Θ The funny thing about it all was that Aset's creative talents seemingly came as a double-edged sword. For as much as they benefited her, they tormented her. With what she painted she simply didn't have the benefit of ignorance when it came to affairs of the heart and in that respect Aset felt that was her curse.

Θ Though, after Jalil Aset still kept her heart open despite the hurt. She knew that soon love would find it's way back to her and so when it appeared as Siris she identified it as such right away. She had even seen *that* in one of her paintings.

Θ Before she had even met Siris she painted him. In fact, it was a painting of both of them together. So when she met him the day on the train she didn't know exactly *how* they would meet again, but she knew that they would and therefore she anxiously awaited the day.

So as she got to know Siris her heart began to open up more and more. Thus, when it came to choose, ultimately Aset decided that once down the road with Jalil was more than enough and if it didn't work the first time than it simply was not meant to be. Besides that she just didn't feel she could ever trust him again for what he had done.

So she went forward with Siris and never looked back. Once she made her decision, Aset and Siris were a match made in heaven, at least that's what she thought. It wouldn't be until well over a year later that Aset would fully appreciate the truth of the nature of their relationship.

5

As she rode on the train Aset recalled how strategic Siris had been in choosing to divulge various bits and pieces of his life to her. Specifically, she recalled how it took him over a month to finally share with her an intricate part of his life story. It was the same life story of many other Carbo men their age.

One evening as they sat watching a movie Si shared with Aset that he was a single man who had never been married, but had fathered several children by several different women. Aset was a bit disappointed, but wasn't surprised by this news because it had become a common story among Carbo men. Though Aset had somehow avoided getting tangled up in the web of it, it had recently become an epidemic that was infecting the Carbo race like the plague. From the perspective of the men it was like some sick sort of badge of honor that they all wore with great pride.

As Aset listened on Siris expressed that though he started young, he was proud to have fathered each of his children. To him they were the evidence of his godhood as it was how he proved to the world just who he was. He said that specifically it was his sons that demonstrated this. According to Siris only God could reproduce himself. So despite their many shortcomings Siris took great pride in his sons.

Siris went on to share with Aset that he had four children by three different women. His oldest two were girls of two different women and his two youngest were boys by the same woman with whom Siris had the longest relationship. He then disclosed that with the exception of the eldest child there were quite a bit of love triangles between the last two women. Siris was still with the second born daughter's mothers when he started seeing the mother of his sons. In fact, the two women knew one another prior and so there was quite a bit of animosity between the two of them.

Then even after Siris started seeing the mother of his sons exclusively Aset gathered from what Siris said that it still wasn't so 'exclusive' because Siris was still seeing his second born daughter's mother on the side along with some other random women. Ultimately, it was Si's cheating that led to the end of his relationship with his sons mother. In her attempt at getting revenge she too started to venture outside of the relationship and it was more than Siris could bear.

After listening intently Aset decided that like everyone Siris had quite a colorful life story for which she would not judge him. Despite what he'd shared with her of it she saw potential in him as a person so she decided to continue to explore things further with him to see where they ended up and so she did.

As time went on and Aset was introduced to Si's children she found it easier to accept things for what they were with Si, at least that's how she saw it. At either rate by the time Aset came along most of Si's children were near if not already into young adulthood. Both daughters were adults and neither cared much to establish a relationship with Aset so whenever they came together it was tolerable at best.

As for the two sons who were in their pre-teens, the relationship was strained from the start because they still had hopes of their parents reconciling. In the eyes of Si's beloved sons Aset would never be welcomed. Though difficult to deal with it was something that Aset eventually came to accept and not take personally. It did, however, tend to sometimes challenge her interactions with Si who would always defended their rude behavior.

To say the least, Aset and Si had a tenuous relationship. Yet, there was a lot about it that Aset absolutely loved. Despite the number of children he had Si was a great father. He responsibly took care of each of them and was very actively involved in their lives. To Aset, Si was affectionate, generous and could often be a lot of fun. At any given moment he would be down for anything and what she enjoyed most about their relationship was how much fun they had together. Besides that Si spoiled her rotten in the way that she was used to being treated.

Yet, Si had another side that wasn't always so pleasant to be around. Once the honeymoon phase faded away this side of Si brought on aspects of their relationship that Aset was not so fond of.

Thinking about this, as Aset rode on the train, she recalled a conversation that she and Siris had regarding a touchy topic just the day before. She was quite taken aback by his opinion on the matter and was still fuming from what he said.

"I agree with the brothahs. The ratio of women to men is currently 4 to 1. On top of that many of the brothahs are locked up or gay so where does that leave the women. I feel like it's something that needs to be settled and polygamy is the best solution," Siris said blankly.

They were both lounging on the couch at Aset's place having one of their intense philosophical conversations. Aset couldn't believe her ears. She'd recently began to notice a change in Siris. She noticed him checking out other women when they went out. In addition to that she was beginning to see the same changes in his behavior that she had seen in Jalil just before he spent the weekend with another woman. So as she listened to him it was like deja vu.

She slowly looked over at Siris and replied, "Oh say it ain't so. Not you! So you want to be with other women. I guess it is every man's fantasy, but I'd expect that to be the case for the *average* man, not YOU!"

"Now see it's not even like that. It's not about the sex. It's about all these women out here that end up being alone in these types of situations when they don't have to be," Siris said.

"Oh it most definitely *is* about sex. So tell me would you take on a second or third wife that was busted?" Aset asked giving Siris the *serious* side eye.

There was too long a silence so Aset answered before Siris could, "Exactly! So it is very much about the sex. Who do you all think you're fooling? And the sistahs claiming to be down with it are full of shit too! I just heard this lame ass sistah the other day talking that mess. Talking about we need to become polygamist for the same tired ass reasons you just gave and because she's tired of sistahs giving her the side eye when they see her with her man and that those of us who aren't down are being childish, selfish and immature. Well guess what I'll be that over this bullshit ya'll are talking. I am not convinced. Ya'll got to come a whole lot better than that," Aset said briefly pausing to readjust herself on the sofa.

Then continuing she said, "First of all, nature takes care of the numbers. There may very well be a lot of brothahs getting killed and locked up, but there are also a lot of sistahs marrying other races and increasingly more who have become lesbians and still several others who have chosen celibacy. So that takes care of the ratio argument. Second as for the jealous sistahs. Well guess what? If they are jealous ass birds *before* they are a co-wife they are gonna be jealous ass birds *after* and will do nothing but come into that household and wreak havoc! I would never bring a jealous ass bird into my home. That's taking one problem and making it another! She'll be jealous every time you spend time with me or if we have children, then if you do for those children and not hers she'll be jealous and will make her kids the same way or she'll just be jealous of the children and the list goes on and on. So no thank you, I'll pass," Aset blasted off.

Siris looked around as if he couldn't believe that he was dumb enough to even broach such a volatile subject. Meanwhile, Aset continued blasting off.

"Now then let us explore the subject of common practice. First of all, even among humans. there has only ever been ONE queen! We both know why. To have it any other way would be an open invitation to total chaos.

Multiple women creates unnecessary imbalances, which creates unnecessary problems. At the end of the day nature, unlike man-made bullshit always takes care to work out imbalances. Man only looks out for his own self-interest and right now you brothahs are spouting a bunch of self-serving bull that I ain't buying!" Aset said fuming.

Siris sat watching Aset in shock as she continued to get more and more worked up. He let her continue because he really didn't have a good enough come back to refute her.

"All these reasons for polygamy that you all are giving are actually *problems* that we need to be finding solutions for. Yeah there *are* a lot of brothahs getting killed and locked up. So what ya'll gonna do about it?!?!!! Ya'll just gonna sit on the sidelines waiting to get their girl when the brothah *does* get locked up instead of doing something to stop it from happening in the first place? Maybe if the latter was the *real* focus then there *would* be enough brothahs out here for the sistahs who don't have one. Your focus is misdirected and you want to tell me that this isn't about sex! Bullshit!" Aset said sternly though still in a calm voice.

She then cleared her throat before continuing saying, "Then back to the point about the sistahs being jealous of the ones that have significant others. Bringing them broads in your house doesn't change the fact that she is a jealous ass bird! What needs to be dealt with is why her ass is a jealous ass bird! Maybe she needs to get some counseling on that and find out why she's like that. Maybe that's why she's alone in the first place. She probably has that issue and a whole host of others that brothahs don't want to be bothered with. We have some serious issues in our community that need to be *addressed* and not brushed under the rug of polygamy! Cause truth be told THAT'S why we're in this mess in the first place. *Who* said polygamy worked before or even now for that matter? Is it real quality sistahs saying that it works for them or is it the brothahs and their groupie minions who are singing its praises? And if it worked so well in the past why was it abandoned? Seems to me your dear old polygamy failed to address the root of the problem even then!"

"Wow you really have some serious opinions about this! I see what you're saying, but I just feel that at the end of the day it's the man's nature to be with more than one woman. One woman cannot physically satisfy all of a man's needs.   That's a natural fact," Siris replied.

"What?!?!! Oh I can't believe this. I can't believe you.   I never would have suspected. Wow!   Hmmm...." Aset fumed before continuing.

"The whole nature versus nurture thing, really?   Well it's funny you should say that because it's a woman's nature to *NOT* want to share her man!   So are we abnormal or defective for being that way?   I think not. Nature doesn't make mistakes. We are made exactly the way we should be.   It's about balance and a man naturally overindulges. It is the woman that teaches him to do things in moderation.   If we allow it, you will do everything in excess throwing off the balance of the entire cosmos. You will eat too much. You'll work too much. You'll sleep too much. You'll give too much. We teach you to balance things out. So in regards to sex you also need to balance that out. Too much of anything can become toxic, the universal law of rhythm tells you that. Sex like everything else in existence must be done in moderation. Not to mention, all that sex with all those women does is exhaust your chi and without that you are nothing! That is your life force energy! You need that to address all of these problems that we're having that we *need* the brothahs to address! But you're too focused on ass to do that," Aset said giving Siris side eye.

"I hadn't looked at it like that, but I guess you have a point," Siris said angling to bring the debate to a close.

"I know I do. You can guess all you want. You'll soon find out. I can show you better than I can tell you," Aset replied.

"What is that supposed to mean?" Siris asked defensively.

"It means that if you're interested in being with other women and you feel that I'm not enough to satisfy you, then by all means please go ahead on. I wish you all the best. I have no desire whatsoever to share my man and I know for a fact that there are plenty of other like-minded brothahs out there who share my sentiments who would be quite fully satisfied with me. Those brothahs know that relationships are about spiritual growth, which means there is no person walking this planet who is going to instantly be everything that you want and completely satisfy you. They know that it takes work and maturity to reach those heights in a relationship. Those brothahs know that HE isn't EVERYTHING that she wants either and he is willing to do the work to become that for her and thus gives her the opportunity to do the same for him!" Aset continued before again shifting in her seat.

Then she looked Siris in the eye and said, "Truthfully you don't even know what the hell you want because you're still growing and learning that about yourself. Yet you expect that a woman, or excuse me, several women are supposed to collectively be so complete when you yourself aren't anywhere near being complete or SATISFACTORY.   Satisfaction comes from within and mature men know that. The more *you* grow in the knowledge of *yourself* YOU begin to fill in the gaps of what you're looking for ro feel like you're missing. As long as you're seeking satisfaction externally you'll never find it.   You know why because your woman isn't the problem *you* are! I look at the brothahs and ask what your external search for satisfaction has gotten you besides fifty babies by fifty baby mommas! Yet, you tell me we're the problem! Maybe those attributes you see lacking in your woman are things that YOU need to work on becoming yourself. So several women is not the answer it's the problem. You need to work on you and if you do that your woman will be all that you desire and more because *you* brothah are magnetic and *you* will then indirectly draw those things out of her unto yourself. She reflects YOUR light and so if the woman in your life isn't all, and I mean ALL that you want her to be perhaps it's because YOU aren't. *You're* supposed to be the All-In-All so when you become that your universe or yoni-verse will reflect that!," Aset concluded before laughing.

"What are you laughing at?" Siris asked seemingly annoyed.

"I'm laughing because none of you has a clue as to who you even are," Aset said before getting up to go to the kitchen to get a drink.

As she walked into the kitchen she couldn't believe that Siris was actually *that* guy. She thought so much more of him. With all of his knowledge of the high sciences she just thought that he knew and understood a lot more.

It annoyed her, even beyond the conversation, because she knew that he was already acting on his opinions on the matter. In fact, she had already seen in one of her paintings that he was already seeing other women. It had come to her clear as day a couple days prior.

Not wanting to relive the heartbreak that she had already experienced in her break-up with Jalil Aset pondered how she would proceed knowing what she knew. She knew that confronting him would do no good because he would merely dismiss what she said as paranoia. She also knew that questioning him would be of no benefit because he would never be honest. So for the time being she settled on keeping it to herself and playing along until she decided what she was going to do and to see how things would unfold.

6

Siris sat on the couch in disbelief at how Aset had reacted to the topic of polygamy. She'd always been quite vocal about her opinions, but never had she spoken to him in so aggressive a tone. He wondered if there was something more to it that she was not telling him. He just didn't understand why she had gotten so heated. She was usually so calm and cool about everything.

He knew that he had done some things, but was careful to make sure that Aset didn't find out so he couldn't imagine why she was responding the way that she was. It almost seemed like she was directly accusing him of cheating. In his mind there was no reason why she should believe such a thing because he did everything to ensure that she always knew that she was his number one. He spent holidays with her, took her around his family and his close social circles. He confided in her about things that he didn't share with anybody else. Most of all he truly did love her. He messed around only as entertainment. Besides that it did a little something extra for his confidence. However, it in no way negated the love that he had for Aset and he more than went out of his way to let her know that. So he really didn't understand where all of her hostility was coming from.

As he sat pondering possible explanations for her annoyance Aset was in the kitchen trying to balance her energy back out. She couldn't believe that she had allowed herself to get so worked up. Usually she kept her cool about things. Even many of the most highly debated subjects didn't get her *that* worked up. She thought to herself that there must have been something between she and Siris that made everything different.

Siris brought out a fire in Aset that she never before knew existed. It seemed the more time she spent with him the stronger that flame within her burned. She decided to ponder it further when she had some time alone to sort it all out and possibly figure out what it all meant.

A few minutes later Siris came into the kitchen asking Aset if she was going to fix anything for breakfast. It was Sunday and going on two in the afternoon and they still hadn't eaten.

"I guess so. We kind of lost track of time on that conversation. I can go ahead now and cook something though," Aset answered while simultaneously getting out some pots and pans to get things started.

"I didn't mean to get you all riled up baby. Whew you were really going in," Siris said with a chuckle.

"Well somebody had to represent for the sistahs that's still being honest about how they feel about the situation. The ones claiming they're down are lying because ain't no woman walking this planet HAPPY about sharing her man no more than a man would be HAPPY about sharing his woman. We aren't THAT different. The same way you all feel about this type of sharing is the same way we feel about it. Why are you all expecting us to be cool and open about something you're not cool and open to. We are a reflection of *your* light so therefore what you're expecting of us ain't natural! You don't want us being with other men so how can you expect us to be okay with you being with other women. *That* doesn't seem natural to me! I'm just not down with spouting bullshit like it's philosophy and on that note I'm done with that conversation. I just thought you should know where I stand on the matter in case you didn't already know. So if that's something you're interested in pursuing you can do so elsewhere with someone else who shares your sentiments and I'll move on with someone who shares mine. That's peace and harmony at it's best and at the end of the day that's what I want for myself and everyone else," Aset concluded.

Siris responded with silence as if still deep in thought and with a look of uncertainty.

Siris tried his best to hide it, but he was deeply bothered by what Aset had said. Based on what she had just said there were clearly things that she wanted that he was not ready to give her and he knew that there would come a day when those things would have to be addressed. He decided that in the meantime he would just enjoy what was and deal with those things when the time came.

Aset made them some breakfast and a couple hours later Siris headed home. She was glad that he didn't stay another night because truth be told after their heated conversation the sight of him was aggravating her. Besides that she needed time alone to sort out her emotions and figure out why they had gone wild.

Once he left Aset sat back down on the couch pondering the state of affairs in her relationship. She wondered how long it would take Siris to snap out of the haze of craziness he was deluded by. Didn't truth and righteousness exist anymore? Why did he and so many other men allow sex to get them so off track?

If brothahs were focused on handling what needed to be handled in the community they wouldn't have time to be so distracted by all that sex with all those women. As far as Aset was concerned time was progress and brothahs were seriously wasting valuable time and compromising significant progress because they were too preoccupied with chasing ass.

She began to see them as a joke and it was becoming increasingly more difficult for her to respect or take any of them seriously! She wondered where the true Gods were? Aset was always an alpha female and wanted nothing more than to be at the side of an alpha male, a true God. It seemed they just didn't exist anymore.

Then, not only were the brothahs no longer alphas, but they had become such hypocrites. Aset pondered, when brothahs started having so little regard for their so-called queens? It was laughable to Aset that they even referred to their women as queens when they clearly had no regard for them as such. If they did they wouldn't have the need for so many other women. In all of history as far as she knew there had only ever been *one* queen whether on a chessboard or ruling a kingdom. So as far as Aset was concerned, just as there was but one king, there was one queen.

Then Aset realized that her annoyance was not just with Siris, but it was with all the brothahs minus the few who were mature and awake enough to see truth. For Aset the union between divine couples was sacred as well as a means for them to collectively change their situation. She realized that she was upset that others could not see that.

In fact, just as that thought came to mind Aset realized that it was the goal of the collective that was the true matter at hand. She decided not to waste anymore of her precious divine energy or mindspace on Si and his childish antics. It seemed that whenever she found herself getting caught up in idle, mundane mind chatter and worry over such things like what Si was or wasn't up to she found that everything else in her life became imbalanced.

So she refocused and redirected her thoughts back to what she needed to do to continue to elevate herself. So as she rode the train reminiscing on the prior day's events she focused inward to try to identify what role she played in creating the debauchery that had become the relationship between she and Siris.

As she began to get her thoughts back on track she asked herself why she even gave a damn? Why did she even care what Si did or with whom? After all she was living her own life which she was always very much in control of so at any given moment she could leave and not have to be bothered one way or another.

She also asked herself why care? Where did caring ever get her anyway? In fact, why was she even being loyal to such an insignificant matter? In the grand scheme of things how much did her relationship with Si really matter? After all, it didn't in any way serve her. It did not match what she desired to have in a relationship so the absence of it wouldn't be any significant loss. Heck, the more she thought about it the more she realized that Siris was taking up way too much valuable space in her thoughts to begin with. She had way better things to occupy her mind with.

So as she approached her stop on the train she brought herself back to that mindful state and her anger toward Siris and all the passengers on the train instantly dissipated. Aset spent the remainder of the day deep in thought about all that was going on with her and what she was going to do to resolve it. She could feel that a thick dark cloud was looming over her. She knew that it would take a great deal of courage and focus to overcome it, but she had faith that she could do it nonetheless.

7

As the day progressed Aset had returned to her normal pleasant disposition. So by the time she got home she felt inspired to paint a new piece, which she called "The Black Wombman Goddess." The inspiration flowed through her paintbrush like a raging river and in no time she had completed what she was certain would be one of her best pieces.

It was a painting of the most compelling perspective of the Carbo woman that she'd ever seen. Aset couldn't believe the magnitude of her own creativity. The Goddess in the painting had glowing green eyes that instantly entranced the onlooker. Physically she was stunning. Then in the background was a penetrating darkness that somehow was nothing and everything at the same time. In a sense the Goddess *was* the darkness, yet on the other hand you could also see that she was an entity that was all on its own. In the distance was what appeared to be a man with a rather covetous expression as he looked on toward the Goddess. His gaze was so penetrating you couldn't help but to obsess over just what he may have been thinking.

To say the least, the painting was quite the conversation piece and Aset couldn't wait to unveil it at her next big showing. She definitely had to reserve this one for the *right* art show. It was sure to turn heads and stir up some conversation.

As Aset stared at the painting she realized how working on it had helped her to come to a decision as to how to handle things with Siris. As was always the case with painting, it calmed her down and gave her a clearer outlook on things. Something about painting was so soothing to Aset's soul. It helped her put things into perspective and see the bigger picture about what was going on in her life. It also enabled her to understand that she was a lot more in control of her life than she thought.

So when Siris called her later that day she was right back to her normal pleasant self as if the heated conversation from the day before had never occurred. Siris was taken aback by her calm demeanor as he was expecting at *least* another few days of her giving him the cold shoulder. He seemingly did not know quite *how* to take her abrupt change in attitude. Either way he decided to go along with it.

"Hey baby, what's going on with you?" Siris greeted warmly on the other end of the phone.

"Oh just thinking about my Si," Aset said sounding dreamy-eyed.

"Oh really?" Siris said surprised.

Siris was more confused than ever. He wondered how things could have changed so fast? Just the day before Aset was striking out at him with a tongue full of nuclear bombs, yet in that moment she was polishing him up with flattery.

"Wow! That's a surprise, but I'll take that," Siris said with a light chuckle.

"So will I be seeing my Si today?" Aset quierried.

"Sorry, but not today baby. I've got some things planned already," Siris answered mysteriously.

"Oh yeah, what do you have planned?" Aset asked.

"Oh just gotta take care of some things. Gonna run out later," Siris answered still being mysterious.

Aset was growing tired of Siris answers that didn't answer anything. She knew that his plans involved another woman, which was why he was being so mysterious. She decided not to question him any further and to instead redirect her focus inward. So she ended the conversation so that she could do just that.

When she got off of the phone Aset tried to figure out why she was so easily taken off track by Siris and his antics. She had already made it clear as to what her position was on being in an open relationship. Furthermore, even in the event that they decided to go their separate ways as a result of it she knew that she would be fine as she always had been.

So understanding why she was so bothered by the whole thing really perplexed her. It seemed a rather mundane matter in the grand scheme of things and Aset couldn't understand why something so insignificant was affecting her in such a significant way.

Aset decided to use her time alone to figure it out. Recently alone time had taken on a whole new meaning for Aset. It seemed every time she was alone the most profound visions came to her. The visions would be so surreal that Aset felt like she had actually transported into them. Moreover, strangely the visions felt like memories, memories that were somehow pieces to a large puzzle. So with each vision Aset became more intrigued and therefore began to look forward to them as she felt that each vision provided her with another piece to the puzzle.

After getting off the phone with Si Aset decided to turn on the television and relax on the couch. She put on one of her favorite home improvement shows and before long a vision came to her.

This time Aset saw what appeared to be some sort of dark Goddess. It was much like the scene depicted in her most recent painting. However, the vision offered Aset a more detailed perspective of things. The Goddess was called Nebet and she had the ability to recall all of her past lives, which was something that seemed all too familiar to Aset. As the vision continued to unfold Aset saw that Nebit was remembering herself as the dark Goddess, wife of Sutekh.

In the memory Nebet was a Goddess who was quite adept at magic. She was particularly good at the art of seduction and sex magic. She longed to have a child, but Sutekh was not ready. He told her that the time was not right and that he still had much work to do in the universe as he was a very powerful and influential God whom many depended on.

Having heard that excuse many times before Nebet was never happy with such responses from Sutekh. Thus, she decided to make some plans of her own as to conceiving.

Nebet was a powerful Goddess of the darkness. In fact, she spent most of her time in a formless state as the darkness. It was how she earned the title, 'Dark Goddess.' However, it was also what made her so cold, ice cold. In fact, it was Nebet who was responsible for bringing about, among the Carbos, what would become known as the return of the Dark Ages.

It wasn't until Sutekh came and illuminated Nebet's dark world that she later came into her true Self. Sutekh brought form to Nebet's darkness and ascribed a proper role and purpose for it. Yet this did not occur until some time later. Prior to that Nebet and her reign of darkness nearly destroyed the dead of the underworld who were the very ones that she had been commissioned to protect.

Sutekh was a powerful God of the heavens. He was known throughout the cosmos as the Illuminated One. Sutekh was also a God of knowledge and as such he held all of the knowledge and secrets of the universe.

For much of their time together Sutekh and Nebet were the perfect balance of light and darkness. They existed in bliss as they complimented one another perfectly. However, as a Goddess of the darkness it wasn't long before Nebet craved more. Her darkness was all-consuming and harnessed a thirst that could never be quenched. So no matter what Sutekh did to please her it was never enough. Nebet could think only of getting more and she began to complain incessantly about it. She also became combative and quite mischievous.

Eventually Nebet drove a wedge so wide between them that Sutekh grew tired and started spending more and more time away from her in the heavens where he kept the company of her sister, Ese.   Soon Sutekh developed a fondness for Ese making Nebet enraged.   It was then that Nebet began to act out of desperation to save her marriage.   She began to use her power of sex magic to appease him, but it was to no avail.   Sutekh had already become disenchanted with Nebet. He grew tired of fighting with the darkness.   He was the Light Bearer and battling with the darkness went against all that he was.

So he began to openly desire Nebet's sister Ese and this made Nebet even more angry.   She got so angry that she decided to get back at both of them by disguising herself as Ese.   Nebet figured that if she looked like Ese perhaps Sutekh would desire her once more.   Her disguise was full proof because even Ese's husband Wasir, who was also Sutekh's brother, was fooled.   This gave Nebet another idea.

Nebet decided that to *really* get back at Sutekh and Ese required the *ultimate* betrayal and that was to bear the child of his brother!

She figured that in doing so she'd get back at Sutekh in the most heinous way possible as punishment for both coveting her sister and for not giving her a child. Essentially, she'd be killing two birds with one stone.

So when the time was right, when Nebet knew that Ese and Sutekh were together she disguised herself as Ese and went to make love to Wasir. Then, as planned, she bore a child fathered by Wasir whom she named Anub. Once Sutekh had learned that his brother, Wasir, had fathered a child with his wife he was outraged and in a murderous rage he brutally killed his brother.

Though as an immortal God Wasir did not actually die, he merely transformed and became ruler of the underworld. So as irony would have it, having been the Dark Goddess, Nebet spent much of her time in the underworld, which meant that ultimately Sutekh's outrage set the stage for Nebet and Wasir to grow even closer. Together Nebet, Anub and his father Wasir ruled the underworld. Meanwhile, Ese and Sutekh grew closer until Sutekh learned that Ese was still in love with Wasir and was secretly still seeing him.

Nebet and all the confusion that she had caused during her fit of dissatisfaction and unquenchable thirst to consume more had successfully cast a thick blanket of darkness over the entire universe and as a result the underworld was bound by havoc and chaos. The light of the Gods had been dimmed to nothingness. This resulted in the Gods going to war with the darkness in an effort to once again reclaim their light.

In the midst of this Nebet was then at the peak of her strength. So as the Goddess of darkness also known as the chaos realm in her anger Nebet casted an illusion that tricked the Gods into voluntarily denouncing their light and submitting to her darkness. This went on for some time and later became what was referred to as the Dark Ages.

Coming out of the haze of the vision and returning back to her own reality Aset realized just what was going on. Her visions were in fact glimpses of her past lives. In that moment Aset felt her past and present as one. It was the centerpiece to the puzzle that connected the entire puzzle together.

Then as if somehow synced up with her thoughts Bast, Aset's twin sister called.

"Hey big sis," Aset gleamed answering the phone excitedly. She was always so happy to hear from her twin. They were identical, but Bast was born a couple of minutes earlier than Aset so Aset always called Bast her big sis.

The two were very close and as children they were inseparable. However, once adulthood hit it seemed their lives took them in different directions. So when Bast started seeing Nigga she moved away to the other side of the country. It was the most difficult experience either of the sisters had ever had. Initially, they called one another all day everyday. More recently, they each began to settle in a bit more into their physical separation calling one another a little less frequently.

They still called one another nearly everyday, but not several times a day unless the other felt that something was troubling the other, which was why Bast decided to call Aset. She felt an emotional disturbance and knew that it was Aset so she called.

"What's going on A?" Bast inquired.

"Girl not much. Just sitting here and got to drifting off again," Aset responded referring to their previous conversations about the recent occurrence of visions of past life experiences that both of them had been experiencing.

Most recently, they both began sharing the same visions and as the same time. When it initially happened they both rushed to call one another only to get the shock of their lives after learning that they both saw the same vision at the same time. More than that they both described an identical emotional experience.

"I know it happened again. I just saw it too. This one was crazy! What really had me buggin was how real it felt this time. It feels more real each time!" Bast replied enthusiastically.

"I know right. What do you think this all means?" Aset asked.

"I'm still trying to figure that out. What I have found out though is that this isn't just happening to us. Other sistahs are getting visions too. They aren't identical to ours, but they seem to also be linked in some way to some sort of past lives like ours. I just saw Iris the other day and she described a horrifying vision to me. Oh yeah and while we're on that topic girl I'm about to have a horrifying scene in real life here with Nigga's ass. Recently he has really been showing himself. I mean girl he's just been all up in everybody's ass. I'm not sure what gave him the impression that it was okay to be so disrespectful to our relationship, but he's about to find out the real deal...." Bast fumed.

"Giiiiirrrrrlllll I'm going through the same exact thing with Si's ass. I don't know what's going on with him either. Like you I'm 2 seconds from being on my way. Then I swear he's lying about something and I feel like it's something big," Aset interrupted unable to contain herself.

"Hmph well I hate to say it, but you already know what he's lying about. For whatever the reason you're just hell bent on him having to admit it to you. Ain't no woman gonna be in no 14 year relationship with a man without him marrying her. You know that baby mama is actually wife. Sis I think you need to to count your losses and move on. I mean how disrespectful to you to lie about something like that. More than that it totally limits the nature of your relationship. I mean how far can it actually go? Unless his status changes he'll never be able to go the distance with you. Hell I feel like that's just how he wants it and truthfully I don't believe he has any intentions on changing it. You deserve better in my opinion. In fact, we both do. I don't even want to get into all that this fool has lied about. I'm in a semi good space right now and I don't want to spoil it by even getting into that. Anyway, we both just need to make preparations to do what we both need to do. I know it and so do you," Bast instructed.

"I'm already with you on that big sis and that's exactly what I'm doing. I'm so ready to do just that. Speaking of which, you should see this painting I just did. It is going to blow your mind!" Aset shared.

"Oh wow! I can't wait to see it. Is it from one of our visions?" Bast asked.

"How did you know?" Aset asked before answering her own question, "Oh yeah, why did I ask that. Of course you know. Yeah as a matter of fact it is. It's the most recent vision we just had, but check this out. This time I painted it *before* having the vision!" Aset said.

"What!?!!? Wow! That's never happened. I wonder what that means," Bast pondered.

"I don't know I just go with the flow of it. I'm sure it will all start to make sense soon," Aset answered sensing a shift in Bast's energy.

"Do you have to get off of the phone big sis?" Aset asked knowing the answer.

"Yeah sis. We'll talk later. Love you," Bast said rushing off of the phone.

"Love you more big sis!" Aset replied.

Aset could always tell when Nigga came around and Bast could no longer speak freely so she'd always end the conversation so that Bast could avoid the awkwardness as Bast always extended her the same courtesy.

Nigga was a very self-absorbed guy much like Si was at times. In both cases both men at times had a tendency to be a little jealous of the sister's relationship. They both acted as if it was supposed to be about them 24 hours a day every time the sisters talked. Neither directly said that, but their negative disposition strongly suggested it.

Si would often act like he was heading out whenever he was around when the sisters spoke and Nigga would act like he needed Bast's help with something every time acting as if her talking to her sister was holding things up. So over the years the sisters had grown accustomed to calling one another when they had a moment away from their significant others.

After she hung up the phone Aset sat and pondered what her sister had said about making a decision about Si. She knew that Bast was right, but she wasn't yet in the right mind space to even deal with the issue and so she didn't.

Aset was confident in her own ability to make the determination as to when the time was right. So she decided to go with her own gut on the matter. In the meantime, she just wanted to enjoy the rest of her time alone doing what she enjoyed, which was watching her favorite home improvement show and daydreaming about the life that was to come for her once she realized her dreams of owning a beautiful home like the ones she saw on the show. So she did.

8

Later on as Aset sat deeply engrossed in her favorite television show with her cat Winter cuddled beside her there was a knock on the door. She wasn't expecting anyone since Siris said that he wouldn't be over so she had no idea who else it could have been. When Winter heard the knock at the door she took off running into hiding.

Winter was a 3-year-old white Persian cat that Aset had adopted a year prior from the Humane Rescue Alliance. Winter was an adorable addition to Aset's household and Aset always said that it was Winter who made her life complete. From the moment they met Winter and Aset were a match made in heaven. Like Aset, Winter was laid back, liked to cuddle and at times had a tendency to be a little high maintenance. Since they were so much alike they understood one another and showered one another with love.

Together Winter and Aset lived in a cute 1-bedroom apartment located in the city in Northeast D.C. off of 4th and H Streets. Her apartment wasn't too far from the Union Station metro and was convenient to all of the downtown shopping hot spots. Aset had her apartment furnished in a modern, cultural theme. Her couch was covered in a conservative kente cloth. She also had a black chaise that sat adjacent to the couch. Aset was really into feng shui so there was no furniture with sharp edges. Her dining table was a cute glass round table that seated four, which had dark tan chairs that complemented the kente cloth pattern that was on the couch tying the rooms together.

Aset had quite the green thumb so there were at least 15 plants all throughout the apartment, which gave the space a cozy feel. Her apartment was on the third floor and got lots of sunlight, which allowed her plants to thrive. Aset decorated her bedroom in earth tones with candles everywhere giving it the feel of a spa. Then throughout the apartment was all of her artwork, which ultimately gave it a gallery feel.

As she got up from lounging on the couch she wondered if it was her friend Tisha who was notorious for popping up on Aset whenever she went shopping at Union Station mall. Aset went to the door and peeped out of the peephole to find that her guess was correct and it *was* Tisha at the door.

"Hey girl!" Aset greeted as she swung the door open to greet Tisha with a warm hug.

"Hey girl!" Tisha squealed back in her high pitched voice.

"What are you doing over here? Spending money as usual?" Aset asked.

"Girl I had to take this bag back that I bought. I ended up not really liking it. For the price I just didn't feel like it went with enough of my outfits," Tisha answered taking her shoes off by the door before heading over to the couch to join Aset who had plopped back down on her still warm spot.

"Well I don't know how that's the case with the amount of shopping you do. You must have an outfit for every purse in existence by now," Aset said jokingly.

"Girl stop. I don't shop that much. When I do it's because I deserve it. I work hard so I should be able to shop hard," Tisha defended.

"Must be nice," Aset said sarcastically before continuing. "So anyway how's it going? And can I get you something to drink while you tell me?" Aset asked.

"Yeah girl. Do you have some wine? A nice red if you have one," Tisha answered.

"I sure do. Now if you're feeling spicy I have a nice Syrah. I also have Cabernet or Merlot if you're feeling more chill," Aset offered.

"Wow! That's a tough choice. Hmmmm…." Tisha said pondering the thought.

Aset got the corkscrew out while Tisha decided which she wanted.

"Ok I"ll take the Merlot please," Tisha answered.

"Great choice. This one is really good too. Si and I picked it up at a wine tasting we just went to a couple of weeks ago," Aset said.

"Oh yeah! Why didn't you tell *me* about it. Eric and I would have loved to go. We love wine tastings!" Tisha exclaimed.

"I'll remember that and let you know if I hear about another one. By the way how is Eric?" Aset asked.

"Umph. Girl we ain't even speaking right now. He is getting on my last nerve!" Tisha complained.

"Girl you always say that," Aset observed.

"Naw girl we *really* got into it this time. We haven't even said one word to each other for over a week now," Tisha said.

"Really! Girl what is it this time?" Aset said coming into the living room with two glasses of Merlot.

"Thanks," Tisha said taking her glass from Aset's hand, "cause I'm gonna damn sure *need* a drink before I get into this."

Aset laughed anticipating Tisha's overly dramatic rendition of what transpired between she and Eric.

"Girl I just get so sick of his ass. I'm doing everything around that house. He doesn't help out with the kids. I'm doing all the cleaning, all the cooking, homework and baths for the kids. I mean I work everyday just like he does and besides that I would just think that he would take more of an interest in being more active with his sons," Tisha complained.

Aset was used to these complaints from both Tisha and several of her other friends. With all of them it was the same grievance. They all felt under-appreciated by their men. They felt that the recognition that their spouses gave them just didn't measure up to all the work they put in.

Aset, who was the only unmarried one among them could never relate to the endless banter and lack of gratitude. To her it seemed that no matter what their spouses did it was never enough. Aset felt that they all failed to see things from their husbands point of view. The husbands saw their contribution as their working hard to financially support the household. So they didn't see a need to also do any of the domestic chores.

Furthermore, in each case their husbands were the primary providers in that they, for the most part, paid mostly all of the household expenses. Thus, for that reason Aset often had a difficult time understanding what there was to complain about. She'd always had to pay all the bills herself. She had to do all the household chores on her own and because she and Siris did not live together many times she ended up doing household chores in both apartments, essentially maintaining two homes. Nonetheless, Aset listened on attentively as Tisha continued her tantrum fussing about all of the things Eric *wasn't* doing.

"Besides that he doesn't even compliment me anymore. I mean it's pretty bad that I have to get compliments from strangers on the street and co-workers. Girl this time we really got into it and I'm seriously considering leaving. I can't take it anymore. That's why today I said I'm gonna go to the mall and treat myself to something. I need that for me. It's always about everybody else and it's never about me," Tisha continued.

"Hmmm. Well girl maybe he just has a different way of contributing to the household. Maybe he considers what he does financially as his way of contributing. As for complimenting you maybe he feels like he *is* doing that by way of the lifestyle that he gives you. Especially by paying all the bills and allowing you the freedom to spend your own money the way you want," Aset offered.

"Girl please. That's bull!" Tisha said as she took a sip of her wine, "He used to compliment me all the time, telling me how beautiful I was and saying how sexy I was. Yet now all I get is his arrogant ass acting like I'm supposed to worship the ground that he walks on because he pays all the bills. I'm supposed to just deal with his nasty ass attitudes and his slick ass remarks. Girl I'm sick of it! I don't care what he's paying. That doesn't give him the right to treat me like shit! Plus I'm just not feeling him anymore. I feel like I'm just going through the motions staying in this marriage. I mean damn is this all there is? Am I just the in-house ass, the nanny and the damn maid?" Tisha asked.

"Well girl, your *all* is a whole hell of a lot to somebody like me who has never had that. Trust me, you don't want to be out here in this dating world. It's not at all that it's cracked up to be. And all that attention you're getting from guys on the streets.... girl do not be fooled! That mess does *not* last and it's only to reel you in. It's all a front. Believe me you're better off where you are. Eric is a good man. At least he *does* take care of his family. There are a lot of guys out here who don't," Aset counseled.

"Yeah well that's not good enough. I feel like there has to be more out there for me than this. I feel like I'm just the damn housemaid with benefits because that's how he treats me so that's the extent of my worth to him. I know for a fact that there are other guys out here that would see me as much more," Tisha said as if hinting around to something more.

"Oh yeah. Well girl don't believe the hype because like I said dudes out here will *tell* you exactly what they know you want to hear," Aset said.

"Hmph. I hear you," Tisha grumbled taking another sip of her wine.

"Girl hang in there. I'd hate to see another Carbo family destroyed. You two can get through this," Aset encouraged.

"I don't think so because I am two seconds away from exiting stage left on his ass. Anyway I don't want to talk about his ass anymore. So moving on....guess what?" Tisha said slyly.

"What?" Aset inquired skeptically.

"Well..... there's this guy that just started working at my job," Tisha said smiling ear to ear.

"Ok and...." Aset pryed.

"Well….. he's someone we both know from Blair," Tisha hinted.

"From Blair? Oh yeah, who?" Aset asked curiously.

"Girl do you remember Brian? Brian that used to have a huge crush on me," Tisha asked.

"Vaguely. I sort of remember his face, but I can't remember that much about him. Anyway, so he's working there now? What does he do?" Aset asked.

"He's an architectural engineer. Still smart as ever. Still sexy as ever and girl I don't know what has come over me, but I am just so giddy around him. It's like everytime I see him I'm right back at Blair. He is still so much fun. He always *could* make me laugh. Remember that girl?" Tisha asked still smiling like she was on cloud nine.

Rolling her eyes upward and shaking her head Aset said, "Sounds like you're treading in dangerous waters."

"Girl so what if I do? Even if I do I will be well within my rights after what Eric did. I'm trying to move on from that, but I don't think I ever will," Tisha said referring to Eric's prior extra-marital affair that he had with a female friend of a couple they both socialized with.

"But girl you said that you both worked through that already, which means that you can't keep holding it over Eric's head. I get that you're not going to just *forget* about it, but either you *forgive* him or you don't. It's not fair for you to say you forgive him, but then proceed to act based on your lack of forgiveness," Aset offered.

"Maybe I could do that if his arrogant ass wasn't acting like *I"m* supposed to put up with all this crap from him when *he's* the one who betrayed *my* trust not the other way around! You would think he'd be more humble and apologetic about the shit!" Tisha said beginning to get worked up as she started to re-live the infidelity.

"Girl I thought he *did* apologize. How many times are you going to make him apologize? At some point you're gonna have to accept his apology or admit to him that you can't. You can't keep pretending to do one thing while feeling something completely different. On top of that now you're entertaining Brian. I'm your girl so I'm gonna keep it 100. That's some foul shit," Aset added.

"I know girl and I'm trying, but part of me feels like maybe if I get with Brian I'll feel vindicated. I was loyal to Eric, a faithful wife, a good mother to his children, a good daughter-in-law to his mother and I used to worship the ground that he walked on and then he cheated on me anyway. How do you just get over that? Tell me how am I supposed to feel motivated to be all of that for him again when despite having done all the right things in the first place he still cheated?" Tisha asked.

As Aset listened to Tisha she thought about her own situation with Siris. She had in every way been a model girlfriend to him, cooking for him, cleaning his house, being faithful and loyal and yet he was still cheating on her. Aset asked herself the same question that Tisha was asking her.

Quickly bringing her focus back to Tisha's situation Aset answered, "You simply remind yourself that there are two people involved in the relationship. Therefore, in some way you played a part in the breakdown of that relationship. Acknowledge that. Forgive yourself then forgive him and take it one day at a time. But I guarantee you that getting involved with Brian is not going to put a band aide on it and make it better. If anything it's gonna make matters worse, especially if you get caught. Don't risk that girl," Aset advised.

"Well trust me I'm not gonna get caught. We're not sloppy like they are. When I'm with Brian I feel so free. I'm always the one at home with the kids and so when I'm with Brian it's a break from all of that. It's a break from being mom. It's a break from being the unappreciated wife. It's a time when I'm the center of this man's attention and sometimes that's just what a bitch needs!" Tisha exclaimed.

"I hear you girl, but if that's the case, if you're really that miserable and you don't believe that you can ever be happy with Eric why not just go ahead and get a divorce so that you can see other men without compromising your vows? If not, then maybe express to your husband that that's what you need from him, more attention, more loving gestures and compliments. If you haven't done that it's not fair to hold him accountable and expect him to read your mind. Either way you have a choice and you can deal with this without betraying your husband and your family," Aset advised.

"Yeah I guess you have a point. I'll think about it girl," Tisha said taking the final sip of her wine.

"Did you want some more?" Aset said getting up to refill Tisha's glass.

"No thanks. I actually have to get going. I gotta pick the boys up from baseball practice," Tisha said sarcastically rolling her eyes upwards.

Tisha and Eric had two sons ages 7 and 9. They'd been married for over 10 years. Eric also had a daughter from a previous relationship who was 13 that lived with her mother in Takoma Park, Maryland.

Eric had always been a bit of a sports enthusiast and his sons were no different. So they were involved in quite a bit of sports, which kept Tisha quite busy running them from one practice to the next.

"Okay girl well I'm glad you stopped by and I hope it helped some coming over here to vent. Feel free to come through if you just need to take a moment. At the same time I hope you consider some of what I said," Aset said getting up with Tisha to walk her towards the apartment door.

"I will girl. I'll keep you posted and call me later," Tisha said leaning in to hug Aset goodbye as she whisked out the door.

When Aset closed the door she thought about Tisha's situation and how it related to her own. She definitely understood Tisha's wanting some form of vindication after being cheated on. However, she knew that in the end it simply did not solve the problem.

The root of the problem went deeper than the Carbo men being cheaters and wanting to have an entourage of women. Something led to that and Aset was more interested in identifying what that was and resolving it. So she focused on doing just that. However, doing so proved more difficult than she anticipated as things began to worsen between she and Siris.

9

As the weeks went by Siris began to act more and more suspicious. All of a sudden his phone rang at odd hours of the night well after midnight on weeknights. He began to take more calls in private and ignore more calls when Aset was around. He also ignored more of Aset's calls when she called him. He seemed to have more 'plans,' of which he concealed the details.

On top of that he was all of a sudden spending so much time "with the fellas." He had a best friend named Chris, who Aset knew was dog. He had a new flavor of the week every month or so. He had absolutely no respect for women and it was evident in his demeanor toward them and even more so in the way that he spoke to them. Aset hated how he'd curse at the women on the phone whenever he came around. It was the one thing about him that just made her blood boil.

Chris also had this really sly look about him that Aset simply could not stand! She didn't even like his main girlfriend, Joy, who Siris and Chris would always encourage Aset to build a relationship with whenever they all went on double dates together. For Aset that was never going to happen because that trick was just as rude and disrespectful as her man.

The first time they met and were introduced Joy threw Aset shade. She didn't know Aset nor did she know anything about her so Aset was confused as to what that was all about. So from that day forward it went downhill from there. Besides that she wasn't anywhere near the caliber of woman Aset befriended so it was just a no-go all the way around.

Aside from being a dog what Aset disliked most about Chris was the strong influence he had over Siris. She really didn't care for how close they were. At times they seemed like more of a couple than she and Siris.

They talked on the phone several times a day and Aset swore they must have seen each other just as much. She'd never in all of her years of dating seen two men *that* close. She'd known men to have guy friends who they went way back with and who would have their back, but she'd never seen two guys talk and spend damn near as much time together as *she* spent with her man.

It was like Chris had to keep a tight reign on Siris and in doing so he influenced Siris to do exactly what he did. They were two peas in a pod, misery's company. Like two old women they bitched and complained about the women in their lives vowing to never truly commit to any of them and to merely enjoy what they considered to be their "blessings," which were the women they had on the side who supposedly 'happily' sat on the bench anticipating their chance to play.

As far as Aset was concerned she truly didn't see them ever committing to any woman because they were already so committed to the monogamous relationship that they had with one another and NO woman was ever going to come between that. It was the most strange relationship she'd ever witnessed between to grown ass men and it sickened her.

Aset wasn't sure if it was their immaturity that annoyed her or their delusions of grandeur, particularly when they were together. Either way Aset was over the recent 'guys night out' rendevous that had Siris leaving her alone on weekends only to come over at 5 in the morning like she was the after party.

Meanwhile, Aset continued to observe the changes in Siris and the more she did the more they confirmed what she already knew. Nonetheless, Aset decided to continue to play along and avoid any type of confrontation while she worked out her plans on how to deal with Siris. However, the more Siris acted shady the more Aset gravitated toward ending the whole relationship and moving on with her life. The reality was that she was really just waiting for a time that was most optimal for her and caused her the least, if any grief.

Aset was a firm believer that ending a relationship was not something that had to result in a long drawn out episode of sadness and heartache. It was never her practice to do so and she was not about to make it so with Siris. So her remaining in the relationship was always about her and never him. When leaving felt good she would do so. It was all just a matter of time and she felt most certain that it was going to be sooner rather than later.

After Tisha left Aset returned to her spot on the couch and put on a movie then drifted off into a deep sleep. It wasn't a normal sleep. It was different in that it seemed to be a joining of the minds of sorts. Aset could sense a connection with Bast, but she also felt a connection to an even larger presence. Besides that it was a resting state, but somehow simultaneously it felt like a contemplative state.

As Aset lie in rest contemplating what seemed to be another past life vision infused with random thoughts about her current situation with Si came into her awareness. She began to see the many cycles of humanity's evolution like a movie on fast forward until it began to slow down. In that moment Aset became a part of the vision. It was as if she was an actress in a movie that she simultaneously watching. At the same time she didn't feel in control of what she was doing and was behaving in a somewhat scripted way. All that she felt in control of was her thoughts. She felt this because what was happening in the vision was in direct correlation to what she was just previously thinking about when Tisha was visiting.

In the vision Aset was a fierce Goddess whose companion had just cheated on her in much the same way that Siris had. He didn't know that Aset had any knowledge of what he had done nor did she tell him. Instead, she tricked the God into coming down to her dark underworld. Over the course of several millenniums he remained there subdued by her alluring charms as he enjoyed a perpetual state of merging with her.

One day he expressed a desire to return to his light. Having expected it, Aset merely ignored his request and continued to captivate him with the lure of her darkness.

Then determined to escape, the God devised another way to escape. Knowing that he would not be able to manage a physical escape he attempted a different ploy. He attempted to seduce her mind into submission to his will. However, Aset was too smart for the God and saw right through his ploy and thus the end result was chaos!

Forcing her out of her sleep-like contemplative state was a jingling of keys at the door. Aset looked over at the clock and as had become the norm it was after 5 in the morning. Siris was developing habits that were definitely shaping up to be the death of their relationship because Aset was truly on the verge of deading the whole thing. She was just not convinced that he was interested in the type of relationship that she was interested in.

Besides that for the life of her she couldn't understand why a man his age preferred to spend his weekends with a bunch of guys partying at clubs rather than enjoying some grown folks fun in the company of his own mature, fun, loving Queen. He acted like he was still in college or something and Aset was used to entertaining more mature men who enjoyed grown folks fun like traveling, weekend getaways, dinner parties, shows and dining out. Though as she heard Siris stumbling into her room having not even noticed that she was on the couch she knew for sure that he was definitely *not* that guy.

It seemed the more Aset tried to see the light in Siris the more her own darkness surfaced and the more it consumed her. It was like he just couldn't go five minutes on the positive with her.

Aset wanted desperately to see and focus on the good in Siris as she knew there was some. However, he seemed insistent on showing her just the opposite making her attempts useless.

The more Siris pulled his stunts the darker Aset became. She was going to such a descended level of darkness that she was becoming a stranger to even herself. Her thoughts of Siris worsened each day and it was getting to the point where she saw nothing good about him and wondered why she insisted on continuing to torture herself by even being with him.

He became the stench that sickened her to her stomach and the rancorous sight of him repulsed her. There were times that even his presence was a vile pestilence. It was those times that Aset just stayed at her place and told Siris that *she* had plans.

However, the worst times were when she couldn't bare for him to even touch her. It was usually when she knew that he had been with one of his other women and was trying to play it cool as if it wasn't the case. Perhaps it was the lying or maybe it was the insult to her intelligence. Whatever it was it left Aset feeling the worse pain ever. It wasn't so much guilt as it was her being upset with herself for even allowing things to get to that.

As Siris made his way to the bedroom Aset remained on the couch with her eyes closed pretending to be sound asleep as she conjured up the soundness of mind easing her stomach enough to get through the night. She figured that if she could make it to the next morning she was good to go and so she did.

10

The next morning Aset woke up at around 9 in the morning bright as ever. She was feeling inspired to paint so she got up, washed her face, brushed her teeth, threw her hair in a bun, slipped on a hot pink cami and some black leggings then headed to the living room with Winter trailing behind leaving Siris snoring in the bed.

Breaking out her paint and brushes Aset got right into it. Seemingly picking up where she left off the night before still inspired by a vision she'd had Aset painted like someone possessed. She painted as if she was seeing the images on a movie screen. Her hand took on a life of its own with strokes that were as compulsive as they were purposeful.

Aset must have gone on this way for over 3 hours without interruption. She was so deeply engrossed in her painting that she hadn't even noticed that Siris had awakened. As he walked into the living room Winter went to rub against his leg. Snapping out of her trance Aset quickly moved her easel so as to prevent Siris from seeing her painting. She never liked anyone to look at her work until *she* wanted them to see it.

"I know, I know. I'm not going to look," Siris said walking into the living room still groggy. "Just coming to say good morning beautiful."

Then he reached down to rub Winter on the head and said "Good morning to you too Winter."

"Good morning," Aset replied blankly.

Aset really wasn't in the mood to be fake like everything was cool and like she didn't have a problem with his recent weekend escapades. She was more than over it and like a drug addict who's high was blown she was actually quite perturbed that Siris had just ruined her creative flow. So she decided that the fewer words the better.

Siris was used to Aset's 'artistic mood swings' so he learned not to take it personal whenever Aset was short with him. He had not a clue that her aloofness had anything to do with his coming over in the wee hours of the morning.

"Baby I have some running around to do. Plus, I got to meet up with Chris so I'm going to head out and come back through later if that's okay," Siris asked while following behind and kissing Aset on the neck as she walked toward the kitchen.

"Yeah that's cool. I have some things to do as well so that'll work," Aset replied with the same dryness as she had before.

She was so glad that he was leaving because the sight of him was beginning to repulse her. Besides that she was looking forward to some time away from him. She needed to get back in tuned with herself. She needed to refocus on what *she* wanted.

So after Siris left, which was within an hour, Aset was able to do just that. When she did she had the time of her life!

She decided to spend the day out. It was a beautiful, sunny Saturday which Aset thought was perfect for getting out to get some creative inspiration. First she went to Georgetown and enjoyed some nice lunch at a restaurant called Sequoia's that overlooked the Potomac River.

She got a table at the window where she enjoyed watching some kayakers and canoers. As she watched them she decided that after she finished eating she wanted to rent one of the kayaks for herself. It was something that she'd never done, but always wanted to try so she did just that.

The day turned out to be one of the most fun-filled days that Aset had enjoyed in quite some time. She did all of the things that she enjoyed doing before Siris. Since being with him she had somehow lost herself in their relationship and with that many of her favorite past times fell to the wayside. Aset used to enjoy hiking, biking, going to museums and art shows. She enjoyed going to movies, plays, shows and dinner parties. She also loved to travel. However, on the contrary Siris just liked to go to the club and that was about the extent of his fun. He acted like a broke college student or like someone who hadn't been exposed to any of life's treasures.

Washington, DC was filled with fun hidden treasures so Aset could never understand how Siris could be such a bore living in such a fun place. She always told him that there was a lot more to life than scattered asses shaking at clubs.

Nonetheless, that day Aset pulled out all the stops for herself and treated herself the way she liked to be treated. She was enjoying herself so much that people were asking to join her because it seemed like she was having way too much fun alone. They were in awe of her ability to be so entertained by herself.

Aset even surprised herself because she actually had never done anything like that before. So she was just as shocked as everyone else by her new found freedom of enjoying her own company.

After kayaking Aset went to an art gallery that she had been meaning to check out in downtown DC. Then afterwards she managed to cop a ticket to the Alvin Ailey American Dance Theatre that was playing at the Kennedy Center, followed by dinner at an Italian restaurant on Pennsylvania Avenue. By the time Aset wrapped up the day and headed home it was just after 11 that night.

Aset returned home to find a fuming Siris sitting on the couch with the television on.

"Oh wow, what a pleasant surprise," Aset said smiling at Siris as she came out of her shoes walking toward the console to plop her purse down.

Siris was irate and didn't seem the least bit happy to see her. Aset knew that he was upset because she was not sitting around the house all day awaiting his return and she could have cared less. She had just enjoyed one of the most wonderful days of her life with herself and she was not apologizing to anyone for doing so, least of all Siris. So she wisped by, kissed him on the cheek and made her way to the bathroom to relieve herself.

She came back out of the bathroom to find Siris sitting on her bed looking like a little boy whose dog had just died. She was in no mood for his dramatics and she could have cared less about his silent treatment so she went on moving about getting settled ignoring him. If he had something to get off of his chest he was going to have to do so without her inquiries.

She had no interest in asking him what he did that day or how long he'd been at her place. Neither did she care to know why he had an attitude. There had been many a time when Aset had come to Siris' place only to find that he wasn't there. Not only was he not there, but often he wouldn't return until the wee hours of the morning. Then when Aset asked him where he'd been he'd damn near bite her head off, chew it up and then spit it out. With that, Aset had already made up her mind that she would not answer any questions as to her whereabouts.

So she and Siris just sort of worked around one another for a while acting as if the other wasn't there until finally Siris broke the silence.

"Have you eaten? Would you like to go out over by my way to grab a bite then spend the night at my place?" Siris asked with a hint of uncertainty as if he anticipated Aset declining his offer.

"Sure. Just give me a minute to change and I'll be all set," Aset said in her still very chipper mood.

Though she'd already eaten she was up for another light meal as several hours had since passed. Besides that she was up to go to Siris' apartment as she hadn't recently spent much time there.

Like Aset, Siris also lived in the city, but just a different part over in N.W. D.C. just about 20 minutes away from Aset off of U Street. He lived in an older apartment building in a two-bedroom apartment. Since Aset had the nicer apartment they typically spent most of their time together at her place.

However, Aset had recently added her woman's touch to Si's bachelor pad making it more cozy by hanging a couple of her paintings on the walls and framing some pictures of them. She'd also gotten him to purchase a few bath towels, kitchen appliances and bed linen making it feel more like a home. Though despite it all the more secretive Siris became the less welcomed Aset felt in his home so she didn't go over as much. On the other hand, Siris had no problem popping up at Aset's house from time to time.

"Ok hurry up now. The clock is ticking," Si said in his more normal tone and with a more relieved, lighter mood than before as he headed into the living room where he plopped down on the couch grabbing the television remote.

Siris always rushed Aset to get dressed knowing that he had popped up on her without the benefit of advanced notice to give her a chance to get dressed before he arrived. She was used to it though so she didn't fuss with him about it anymore.

Siris had a way of bringing out the spontaneity in Aset. For the most part she was very conservative and routined. So his popup visits made Aset step outside of the box that she lived in.

Within about half hour Aset was dressed and ready to go. She had put on some skinny jeans and a cute lavender sleeveless swoop down shirt that had silver flowers imprinted on the front.

"Wow you look nice. May have to take you out dancing somewhere after," Siris said looking at Aset coyly.

"Is that so," Aset answered. "So where are we going to grab a bite?"

"I was thinking breakfast food at that diner place you like over in Georgetown. That way we'll be close enough to things to perhaps catch a club in time. Is that cool?" Siris said.

"Yeah that sounds perfect," Aset answered grabbing her purse from the console table near the front door.

They both slipped on their shoes and headed out the door to the restaurant. It was mid summer and Saturday night so the restaurant was buzzing. It was a nice night so lots of people were out enjoying the summer air. Aset looked over at Siris and remembered why she loved him so much. He would always do things like that out of blue that reminded her of what he meant to her.

She decided to not think too hard on what had transpired the night before or earlier that day and just allow the evening to unfold. In the meantime, she focused on enjoying the evening out with Siris. So they both did just that. They ordered their food, enjoyed some light conversation and then spent the remainder of their time in the restaurant enjoying the silence of one another's company.

Afterwards, as promised Siris took Aset out dancing. He took her to a spot not far from his apartment that was playing old school hip-hop called the U Street Music Hall. Though it was well after midnight by the time they arrived the club was still jumping and the dj was playing all of their favorite songs.

Like most things Si and Aset also had the same taste in music. They were both old school hip-hop fanatics enjoying artists ranging from Pete Rock and CL Smooth, EPMD and Gang Starr to Nas. It seemed the dj was reading their minds because he was playing all of those artists and some. From the time they walked in the door Si and Aset were jamming so hard that they couldn't pull themselves away from the dance floor long enough to take a break. The way they were acting one would have thought that they were both teenagers again.

As they danced Siris gazed into Aset's eyes as if his love for her had been renewed. She could see in his eyes pure love and it was a look that she hadn't seen in months. As she gazed back at him feeling the same love for him she wondered if perhaps things would begin to improve for them. However, she didn't want to spoil the moment so she just stayed in the present and enjoyed the moment as it was.

They danced the night away all the way up until the club lights came on. It ended up being one of the most beautiful nights they had in a long time, at least until it wasn't. Just when the evening couldn't get any better things took a turn for the worst.

When the lights came on Aset noticed that a woman a few feet away from them near the bar had been staring very intensely at them. Aset knew that look anywhere. She knew from the woman's gaze that she knew Si. More than that she apparently thought that whatever was going on between them was more than just casual at least she wanted it to be.

Aset knew that this was merely confirmation of what she already knew Siris was doing so she tried to keep herself calm and not even let herself get all worked up.

The woman was dark-brown skinned with short hair. She was a couple inches taller than Aset and quite a bit thicker than Aset. As Aset looked at the woman she was somewhat

Black Wombman

taken aback because the woman wasn't very attractive. Besides that she had no idea that Siris was even into big girls especially given the hard time he gave her about keeping her body in shape. At the slightest hint of some stomach fat he would start throwing her hints, buying her workout equipment or sending her workout videos. So Aset was surprised to say the least in Siris' apparent change in taste.

Siris had not yet noticed the woman staring, but Aset could feel from the weight of the woman's stare that she did not plan to let Si leave without making her presence known. So Aset calmly and patiently waited.

"I just need to run to the bathroom baby and then we can head out," Si said yelling over the music in Aset's ear.

"Ok I'll come with," Aset said trailing behind him. She knew that if she allowed him to walk to the restroom alone the woman would have likely confronted him privately and there was no way that she was going to let Siris off the hook that easy. It was time for them to discuss the issues out in the open. Besides that she was tired of wondering where things stood with them and was happy to finally have the opportunity to get some resolve regarding the matter.

So as Si made his way into the restroom Aset stood nearby keeping the mysterious woman in view. Aset wondered what he had told the woman. She figured that he was probably up front with her having informed her that he was in a relationship along with a list of complaints. Men usually told the 'other woman' about their main woman so that she knew not to have any expectations of things getting serious between them or in the event of a chance encounter to ensure that she did not make a scene. Yet, this approach never truly worked because women could never *truly* refrain from getting attached. Moreover, they *always* had their own hidden agenda of proving him wrong, trying to win his affections in an effort to earn the top spot.

So Aset was more than certain that this woman had it set in her mind to do just that as she still felt the intensity of her stare. People were beginning to clear out of the club by the time Siris came out of the bathroom and Aset noticed that the woman was still hanging around no doubt waiting for the opportunity to make her presence known to Siris.

Siris grabbed Aset's hand and they headed toward the exit. Then as expected as they made their way to the door the woman walked in front of them just as they were making their way through the doorway.

Giving him a huge smile she looked at Siris then Aset and said, "Hi Siris! What a surprise seeing you here. How are you?"

After a momentary flash of shock then struggling to appear in control Siris calmly answered, "Hi! I'm good just out enjoying the nice summer night." Then looking at Aset he said, "Forgive me, Aset this is Ujana, Ujana this is Aset."

Extending out her hand to greet the woman Aset said warmly, "Peace Ujana, nice to meet you."

With a cold catty reply Ujana replied with a mere head nod then went on to speak to Siris.

Staring at him intensely she said, "Hmmm so what are you getting into now? Heading in?"

"Yeah I am, but it was good seeing you. Take care," Siris said grabbing ahold of Aset's hand slightly tighter privately signaling to her that they were leaving.

Ujana narrowed her eyes at Siris being sure to make him aware of her annoyance.

"Well it was nice meeting you Ujana," Aset said smiling as she turned to leave with Siris.

That made the woman even more irate. She rolled her eyes at Aset as she stood still frozen in disbelief at having seen Siris there with her.

As Siris and Aset walked down the street Aset asked half grinning, "So you wanna tell me who that was babe? It's clear that something is going on between you two. I mean the shade and all the eye rolling made that quite obvious."

"Babe that was nothing. Someone from the past. You know how you all are when we move on," Si answered.

"Oh is that what it was?" Aset said laughing. "Well from the look on her face that looked real fresh to me. I also know how we are when we know you're juggling but aren't being real with ourselves about it."

"Aset stop playing. Don't even go there," Si said trying to be done with the conversation.

"Right," Aset said smiling.

She knew that Siris would never admit what he was doing. Brothahs would lie about cheating to the grave. She could have caught him in the act of having sex with the woman and he still wouldn't admit it. So Aset decided not to press the issue or probe any further. As far as she was concerned she had taken care to do what she needed to do. She had already made it clear to Siris that she had no interest in sharing him with other women. Besides that she knew that the truth would be revealed in a way that he would not be able to deny soon enough as such things always had a way of working out that way so she decided not to worry about it.

Though shifting back to the mood that she was in before seeing the woman proved quite difficult. It wasn't until they had made their way back to the car that Aset was finally able to turn the tide on her thoughts and mood. Ironically, it seemed even more difficult for Siris to do than it was for her. For a while Siris was very quiet during the walk back, seemingly deep in thought. In fact, he didn't break his silence until they got halfway to his place. Aset suspected that he was no doubt reeling internally while trying to maintain a cool exterior and blaming Ujana for *his* getting busted. He was infamous for blaming his screw ups on the women in his life.

"So I want to be with you. You sure you don't mind if we stay at my place tonight?" Siris asked.

"No, not at all. It's been awhile since I've been there. I wasn't sure if my privileges had been revoked or not," Aset said half-jokingly attempting to lighten the tension.

"Oh come on now. You know it's not like that. We've just been chilling at your place more. I thought you liked that.... you know being in *your* space for a change. It's good to balance it out don't you think?" Siris asked.

Aset didn't answer and merely rode the remainder of the way to Siris's house in silence. As they rode along he grabbed ahold of Aset's hand seemingly deep in thought again.

When they arrived at Siris' apartment he lit a few candles and some incense. It was clear that he wanted to set a romantic mood. As bothered as Aset was by his recent behavior Aset figured that the knocking around of flesh and bone wouldn't do any more damage so she decided to go along with it. Besides that it was during sex that Aset could read him best and she needed to get a read on where Siris truly was with things. That night Siris made love to Aset more passionately than he had ever made love to her before. In return she loved him magically.

As she did Aset envisioned them as the characters in one of her past life visions, as a

God and Goddess. She closed her eyes and saw she and Siris back in a time long ago when she went by the name of Ese she saw herself love Siris with the vigor of the love Goddess she once was.

As Ese she was the queen of sex magic and through her yoni she and Siris manifested the heavens as worldly dominance. As she loved him she took Siris' secrets and morphed them into seeds of dominion, which she scattered across the universe. She loved him back into his godhood that night and in doing so Aset imagined that the two of them changed the entire course of mankind. That night, through her darkness, the sex magic bitch Goddess had awakened herself.

12

Exhausted from the workout the night before Siris and Aset slept well into the late afternoon, not waking up until after 12 noon. Siris was the first to awaken. He looked over at Aset who was still sleeping peacefully. As he watched her he thought about the blessing that she had been to him.

Aset was the kindest, most warm-spirited woman that he had ever encountered. From the day they first met she always treated him with such affection even when he treated her harshly. He felt love from her that he had never felt from any other woman before. He watched her and as he did he saw her begin to glow. She radiated an alluring, iridescent light that somehow pulled him in. So without thinking he reached over and kissed her softly on the lips.

Awakened by his kiss Aset smiled then opened her eyes and said, "Ummm now that's a delicious way to wake up. Good morning love."

"Good morning queen," Siris said smiling back at her.

"How long have you been awake? What time is it?" Aset asked.

"I haven't been up long. It's pretty late though. It's after 12 now," Siris replied.

"What!??!!! After 12?" Aset exclaimed.

"Yeah. Why are you so surprised. That was *some* workout last night," Siris said grinning.

"Yes it was my champion lover," Aset replied jokingly.

"So I'm pretty hungry. Wanna grab some brunch at Sankofa?" Siris asked.

"Yeah that would be great, but I have to see if I have any clothes over here. If not we'll have to swing by my place first," Aset answered.

"You *do* have some clothes over here. It hasn't been *that* long," Siris said sarcastically.

"I'm sorry babe. I wasn't implying that it *had* been. I just wasn't sure if I still had any left here with all the shuffling back and forth we've done," Aset explained.

"Ok. Well let's get cleaned up so we can head out. I'm starving," Siris said hopping up out of the bed to head to the bathroom.

Aset smiled as she looked around. It had been a while since she'd spent time at Siris' apartment. She actually sort of missed being there. Though his apartment wasn't as nice as hers she was proud of how the work that she had put into it had given it a more warm and inviting feel.

The bedroom was basic black, but she had softened it up with grey and white bedding and some throw pillows. Though the changes were seemingly minor they made a world of difference. His living room was much of the same basic black with a leather couch and matching loveseat so Aset livened it up with one of her colorful paintings giving it a less cold look. Since Si insisted on keeping the black color theme throughout his apartment Aset hung a black and gold print shower curtain in the bathroom along with black towels with gold trim.

Siris wasn't by any means neat so the one thing that she disliked about coming over was that she often felt like the maid because she always found herself cleaning in an effort to make herself feel comfortable. Aset was just the opposite so she could never shower or prepare anything to eat or drink at Si's apartment unless things were immaculately clean *and* up to her standards.

While Aset was still laying in the bed admiring her work Siris called out to her to join him in the shower.

"Coming Si," she yelled back in the midst of a big yawn.

"Were you just gonna leave me in here to fend for myself? What happened? You fell back asleep?" Siris asked as Aset walked into the bathroom groggy.

"No I was just daydreaming I guess," she replied.

"Oh yeah, about me?" Siris said matter-of-factly.

"Yeah, you know me so well," Aset answered as she joined Siris in the shower.

"I am in fact the best knower," Si said handing Aset her bath sponge.

They both sponged each other down, rinsed then dried off, got dressed and headed to brunch. Aset considered stopping by her apartment first to feed Winter, but decided to wait until afterwards. She figured Winter should have enough food to tie her over. Surprisingly Siris didn't have a snide remark. He always seemed to have a problem with Aset having to always make provisions for her pet. He wasn't much of a pet person so usually when it came to Winter they usually had to agree to disagree.

When they arrived at the restaurant they were surprised to see that there was some type of event going on. There were artsy looking people everywhere.

"Looks like your kind of vibe queen," Siris said to Aset jokingly.

Siris always had jokes about Aset being an artist. He also liked to make very stereotypical statements about the types of events she enjoyed going to.

"Yeah, funny funny," Aset said looking around. "Should we stay here or go somewhere else. It's kind of crowded."

"It's fine. We're already here now. Besides, I'm starving and whatever is going on doesn't seem to be affecting the restaurant section so we're good. Let's get a seat," Siris said looking around for a good seat.

Sankofa was a bookstore and cafe so half of the space was used as a restaurant and the other half as a bookstore where they often hosted various events. The space was small, but cozy.

At the time there seemed to be some type of film premiere going on so quite a few people were there making the space even more 'cozy.' As everyone began to get settled Siris and Aset listened on to see what the film was about. From the looks of it the film seemed to be about women because there were a lot of women in attendance, more so than men. It seemed the men in attendance were likely just there as a result of being dragged there by their women.

Just as everyone was getting settled Siris spotted a small table that seated two not far from the bar. He grabbed Aset's hand and they made their way to the table then sat down. Then so as not to be disruptive to the speaker who was just about to say something Siris whispered to Aset that he was going to go order them something. Aset nodded in reply then listened on to hear what the film was about as Siris made his way over to the bar.

13

"So first I'd like to thank everyone for coming out to see the premiere of *Black Woman Bitch*. I know that many of you are anxious to see it as the title has stirred up quite a bit of controversy. What I do hope is that you will all watch with an open mind and be ready to receive the message that the movie has to offer. When I wrote the treatment for this film I did so with the mindset that the time had come for us as a nation to awaken to some things that are crucial to what is to come in the very near future. In particular I want the sistahs to really tune in to the deeper message in the movie because there are a lot of nuggets in there for you. With that said, thank you all again for your support and for coming out. Enjoy," a brown-skinned young woman said before taking her seat in the rear of the cafe.

A brothah in the back manning the projector immediately started the film. We all looked on anxiously. Then in the nick of time Si returned with their food. The two of them ate as they watched on to see the film.

The film started out with a dark-skinned sistah rising out of what appeared to be a black mist. She looked to be a Goddess of some sort and as the camera zoomed out onlookers could see her as the moon. She had the most hypnotic glow.

Next the sistah looked over and smiled at what at first seemed to be a bright beam of light. As the camera zoomed in closer the viewer saw that it was a very illuminated brothah who was smiling back at the sistah. As the two of them gazed at one another they began to move in an out of one another almost as if they were becoming one at times.

They appeared so much in love that their love could even be felt by those watching the film. It was a feeling of love that could not be expressed in words, but that the film had captured quite well.

Then abruptly the scene changed and the sistah who had seemingly dreamt the scene before woke up. On screen was a Carbo couple lying in bed. The woman was awake and turned away from the man who was still asleep. It was evident from her body language that she was unhappy.

About a few seconds later the brothah woke up, yawned, stretched then got up, out of the bed without even looking at or speaking to the sistah. He went into the bathroom then came out, got dressed and left without saying a word.

As he was leaving out of the room the sistah mumbled, "Bitch ass nigga! Forget you and don't bring yo ass back in my house again! Them locks gon be changed when you get back!"

He was already out the door by the time she had gotten halfway into her sentence so he didn't hear most of what she had said. The sistah sat upright in the bed seemingly very angry.

As the movie unfolded the character of the sistah became quite disheartening. She was the mother of 2 children for whom the brothah that had just left had fathered. Apparently, she had decided that she no longer wanted to be with him or raise her children so he was raising the children. He had come to her house to ask her for some help with the children and the visit later became sexual.

The brothah was working a dead end job and was barely able to make ends meet, which was why he was asking the sistah for some assistance. In turn, she used her powers of seduction to divert his attention away from the children for a while. Then as seemed to be the case typically he fell for it then woke up later disgusted with himself for having done so which was why he left without saying a word.

The movie went on to show how the lives of both the brothah and the sistah differed. While the brothah spent all of his time working hard, doing his best to raise their 2 small children the sistah was out partying with her single friends, traveling and enjoying her fair share of men as she searched for who she believed would be Mr. Right.

Meanwhile, the film showed that what was going on with the couple was no isolated occurrence. Carbo couples all over the planet were experiencing the same thing. Things had gotten so bad that everybody's woman was sleeping with everybody else's man. There was no loyalty among the Carbo couples. As for the brothahs, they were just as dysfunctional. Even those brothahs who had attentive, faithful women started cheating on them as if guarding themselves in anticipation of future betrayal.

Even worse the sistahs were calling all the brothahs weak bitch ass niggas while the brothahs were calling all the sistahs scandalous ass bitches. It seemed to be that being a bitch whether it was man or woman was the theme of the movie.

The men were viewed as such by the woman because the woman perceived them as weak when they couldn't afford to give her the lifestyle she wanted or because they were what she saw as too sensitive or because she felt she could jerk them around.

The women were viewed as such because they had become cold and hard and were acting more like men. They had lost all of their feminine, nurturing qualities.

Next, the movie showed how ultimately these were all of the factors responsible for destroying the Carbo family. Then the strangest thing began to happen. A dark mist appeared covering the entire planet. It looked to be the Goddess that was shown at the beginning of the movie.

She had expanded to a size far larger than the sun God that she was with. At the same time he took on a less illuminated appearance. As a result, the moon began to fade, the planets started to turn to ice and the stars became so dim that they were barely visible.

Then there were flashbacks of how at one time the stars from light years away could be seen in the night sky on planet Earth. However, as things started to transform, man on Earth could hardly see them without an instrument such as a telescope.

Then things in the movie got even more strange. The more the couples cheated on one another, became more divided and were less attentive to the children the more the Carbo couples began to disappear. Their bodies literally began to disappear and that was how the movie ended.

To say the least based on the crowd's reaction the ending of the movie was very unexpected. Everyone in the bookstore was absolutely speechless as it was dead silent. No one moved and you couldn't really get a read from anyone's facial expression as to what they thought about the film.

Just then the woman who had introduced the film came back up to the front and the brothah turned the movie off and turned on some music that softly played in the background.

By then Siris and Aset were done with their food. However, they hadn't left yet because they had gotten so intrigued by the movie. Like everyone else they were anxious to hear what the woman had to say.

"So I'm sure that you all have a lot of thoughts that you would like to share and I would like to give you the opportunity to do just that. I'll be here hanging out for the next couple of hours and would be more than happy to entertain any comments or questions you may have," the woman said eagerly.

With that the brothah in the back turned the music up slightly louder and afterwards several people got up from their seats to make their way to the lady.

"Wow that was some film!" Aset said to Siris as they both remained seated looking at one another still in shock by what they had just seen.

"It was! I mean based on the title I kind of wasn't sure what the film was about, but it definitely turned out to be quite fitting. Very interesting. She really captured a lot of the essence of what's going on in the community because I know quite a few brothahs who have recently become single parents. That used to be unheard of when we were coming up, but today it's becoming more and more common," Siris commented.

"Yeah, I've been noticing that too. I just saw a friend of mine the other day who was talking like she was headed down the same road as many of the sistahs in that movie. I don't even know what to say about it. I don't know what's going on with us these days," Aset replied.

"Yeah, but this is all by design and sistahs should know that by now with all that we've gone through these past several hundred years. The Carbo man in the United States had been strategically made to feel inferior in every way. He educated himself and that wasn't enough because there weren't but a handful of opportunities that were going to be given to the lot of us. So where does she think that left the rest of us. Then we had to come home to hear her bitching about how sorry we were. How was that gonna motivate him to do what was necessary to change the situation," Siris rebutted.

"Babe I'm not saying I don't understand what's really going on. I do. I am more concerned with directly addressing it for resolution purposes because this battle of the sexes that we're doing isn't getting us anywhere. In fact, what it's doing is making us disappear just like in that movie. We *are* becoming less and less relevant in the world. Hell they practically wrote us out of history. On top of that they've pretty much replaced us in the labor market. They've kicked us out of every major city that we used to dominate forcing us all to disperse into oblivion," Aset replied.

"I agree with that. We do need to *do* something about it and it has to start with the Carbo man and woman. That's the challenge though because we are divided now more than ever. Besides that the majority of us are too far gone and unable to even see what's going on. There are only a very select few of us who *do* know and actually that's all it takes to turn things around. We just have to make some moves that's all. I'm glad we came here today. I guess we ended up here because we were supposed to be here," Siris said.

Midway into Siris' reply Aset had gotten distracted and kind of zoned out. She didn't really hear much of anything that he said. In fact, Aset had pretty much left the building.

Siris noticed and asked with a hint of concern, "Baby is everything okay?"

Aset looked straight ahead with a mixed expression of perplexity and annoyance. Just as Aset was about to respond she looked up and to her surprise an unexpected visitor had made their way to their table. To say the least it was not a welcomed surprised. In fact, it was one that just may have been what finally tipped the scales for Aset.

14

Aset looked on to see that coming towards their table was the woman from the club the night before, Ujana. Ujana's eyes were intensely fixated on Siris and she was looking more irritable than ever. She tried, but was unsuccessful at hiding it.

Aset looked back at the woman just as irritated. She was beginning to get annoyed by the woman. Not only had she ruined a perfectly good date the night before, now she was ruining their Sunday brunch, which happened to be something they hadn't done in quite some time. The woman's constant interruptions were beginning to seriously bother Aset and it was getting to the point that if Siris didn't handle it she was going to handle his ass.

Aset gave Siris a stern look signaling him to get rid of the woman. She was not going to be run off by some random woman and felt that Siris needed to handle the matter once and for all.

"Hi again Ujana. What a surprise bumping into you again. Aset you remember Ujana from before don't you," Siris said politely.

"Yes I do. What a surprise seeing you again. Hmmmph I'd almost think that you were stalking us," Aset said half-jokingly.

"Hi," Unjana said to Aset curtly before directing her attention back to Siris. "Yeah it is a surprise seeing you again. Seems I *keep* seeing the two of you everywhere I go. This was my friend's movie premiere and I was here supporting her. What brings you two here?" Ujana inquired.

"Just came to grab a bite and decided to stay once we saw the movie premiere was happening. But it was good seeing you. We're just gonna continue with lunch. Take care,"

Siris said abruptly making Ujana even more upset.

"Siris may I have a word with you over here please?" Ujana asked ice grilling Siris.

Without delay Siris said, "I'll be right back," as he looked over at Aset warmly then back at Ujana with slight irritation.

Aset was annoyed at having her whole vibe thrown off and her time with Siris interrupted yet again by Ujana. However, she was happy to let him speak to her in private so that he could deal with the matter once and for all.

One would have expected Aset to be threatened by the woman and Siris' relationship with her. Yet, Aset wasn't the least bit threatened. It was clear to her that whatever went on between Ujana and Siris was a fling and therefore irrelevant to what was currently going on between Aset and Siris. She could feel Siris' love for her the night before and even then she could see it in his eyes. Therefore she wasn't the least bit concerned. Besides that the two of them were always able to have very candid, mature conversations concerning such things so Aset knew that they would speak openly about the nature of his relationship with the woman later.

Ujana had walked over near the door where Siris followed her. He could tell from her body language that she was irate. However, he was more angry with her than she was with him. He had more than made himself clear as to the nature of their relationship so he was perplexed as to why she was so angry.

"Who is that?" Ujana said with a hint of jealousy.

"Don't you question me about who I'm with as if it's any of your business. Look I told you at the gate what this was. Don't act like now its a problem. You knew what this was!" Siris said irritably.

"I know what you said, but what was all that spending the weekend with me and coming with me to our family functions, hanging out with me partying and whatnot. You were acting like you wanted more," Ujana said with a hurt look on her face.

"So what! I told you what this was. Nobody told you to let your imagination get the best of you. I'm not with you like that and I don't want to be with you like that. As a matter of fact, this shit is dead and don't do this again. Now I'm not trying to hurt your feelings, but I told you what this was for a reason so that we could avoid this. Now shit is all awkward and it didn't need to be. I'm sorry if you got mixed messages because that was not my intention. However, I think it's best we don't see each other anymore. Good luck with everything," Siris said coldly then walked away without even allowing Ujana to respond.

Ujana stood looking as if Siris had taken a dagger to her heart. His words stung, but there was nothing she could say in response because he *had* told her what it was. So moments later she became angry with herself for being such a fool and letting him play her the way he had. Part of her wanted to confront him in the presence of Aset because after what he had done to her she didn't believe that he should be able to just go on to be happy with someone else as if she didn't matter. Yet, she was too much of a lady to embarrass herself in that way so she held her pain in, put on a brave face and went to mingle with her friends.

Meanwhile, Siris returned to Aset. On his way back he knew that he would be expected to have some form of an explanation for Aset. So he was prepared to simply tell her the truth. He really cared about Aset and valued the bond that they both shared. He did not want to jeopardize losing her. Thus, he figured that in this case honesty was his best option. Besides that he had a feeling that Aset had already figured out what was going on. He knew that she was nobody's fool.

"Sorry about that baby," Siris said coming up from behind Aset greeting her with a kiss on the cheek as he made his way back to his seat. If you're ready we can go ahead and head out. I think this event is about over anyway. I see quite a few people clearing out."

"Sure that's fine," Aset said grabbing her purse from the arm of her chair before getting up to leave.

She knew that what Siris really wanted was to get as far away from the awkwardness of the situation as he could. Though she felt no sympathy for him as he had brought it all on himself.

Nonetheless, as they both headed to the door it seemed they had to walk past Ujana to get to the door. Aset gave Ujana a brief glance as they passed her while Siris passed by without saying anything further. Aset could not *wait* to hear what Siris' explanation would be. She knew that it either had to be the truth or a damn good lie, the latter of which she hoped he didn't dare insult her intelligence with.

The moment they made their way out of the cafe the vibe between Siris and Aset instantly became so tense that you could cut it with a knife. Aset was both anxious and curious to hear just what his explanation would be so she waited for Siris to speak. She planned to let him speak too getting it all out and without interrupting him in the least bit. She already had her poker face ready. As far as she was concerned that conversation was long overdue.

However, contrary to Aset's expectations Siris was dead silent. It seemed they were walking for hours as they made their way back to the car because the silence was as heavy as a ton of bricks.

Aset wondered just how long Siris planned to carry on the silent treatment as if *she* had somehow wronged *him*.

"Is he serious right now????" Aset thought to herself.

She wasn't even sure why she was even surprised. Siris was infamous for doing shit then not addressing it leaving time to allow things to die down so that he could avoid having to address it. However all that ever did was cause issues to build up, which was exactly why he and Aset's relationship was already in the trouble that it was in.

Nonetheless, Aset maintained military silence as she refused to initiate the obviously much needed conversation. He was the one doing her dirty and so he was going to have to man up and own up to it and Aset wasn't about to make that easy for him.   So she quietly committed to making him do just that as they walked back to the car then rode along back to Siris' place in silence.   Then, when they got into the apartment and sat on the couch finally Siris spoke breaking the deafening silence.

15

To Aset it seemed like it took an eternity for them to make it back to Si's house. Yet, to Si time was the one commodity that he at the moment seemed to not have enough of. Nonetheless, as he sat on the couch across from Aset sensing her silent demand for an explanation he nervously, but with confidence began to speak.

Though he knew that the truth would hurt he also knew that it was what he had to do to save his relationship with Aset. Things had been kind of going downhill for them for some time and he knew that it was because *he* had been drifting away. Yet, he was sure that he didn't want to lose Aset so he knew that he needed to do whatever it took to keep her. So once he felt ready as he sat down beside Aset on the couch he looked her in the eye and began.

"Baby I know that you must have questions about who that woman was that we saw both the other night and today. I want you to know that she means nothing. She's someone I knew, but no longer deal with. We both have a past and she is part of mine. I still kept in contact with her and may have seen her once or twice since we've been together, but I was very clear with her in telling her that I was not interested in being with her," Siris explained while Aset looked at him skeptically and taking a long pause before responding.

"So you're basically saying you just know her from the past, but you two aren't sleeping together now? I highly doubt that. Her eyes told me that much. She looked like she had very good reason to think that you two were an item," Aset replied.

"I didn't say that we didn't ever sleep together, but she is the past," Siris answered.

"Ok so now we're going to play word games. You know what I'm asking Si. Have you been sleeping with her recently because I know what I just saw back there?" Aset asked curtly.

"It wasn't all that recent," Siris responded nervously.

"Well how recent is 'not all that recent Si?'" Aset asked.

Looking around more nervous than ever and beginning to take on a more defensive tone Siris said, "Not recent is not recent. It's means exactly what I said."

"Hmmm ok. I see. Well it's clear to me that either you're not ready to speak to me honestly about this or you want to insult my intelligence. Please just be honest Si. I promise I'm a big girl and I can assure you that I can handle it. We've always been able to enjoy a very mature, candid relationship and pretty good communication with one another and this is no different. I really can't stand the lying Si," Aset lectured still managing to maintain her calm.

After a very long pause that lasted at least 15 minutes Siris replied, "Ok you're right. It's been during the time that we've been together and it only happened once. I told her that I didn't want to be with her and that sex was all that it was. She knew what it was so I don't know why she was acting like that back there."

Surprisingly still calm, Aset answered gazing at Siris intensely, "Well first of all thank you for being honest. I get that you explained to this woman that you had no interest in anything serious. However, my concern is not that. My concern is that you disrespected the sanctity of *this* relationship by even dealing with her. It's just like we spoke about the other day. The relationship between Carbo man and woman is no longer sacred. It's no longer divine and it can't be when you are running around here with all of these different women for the sake of boosting your ego, trying to compensate for your apparent lack of self-confidence, because of peer pressure or whatever the other ridiculous reasons there are for why you do it."

Before continuing Aset paused briefly and just stared at Siris who was vexing and sulking at the same time on the couch.

"I have done everything in my ability to be all that you have expressly desired in your queen. More than that I have *never* stepped out on you and I never would because I respect you and this relationship too much. You brothahs claim you cheat because women aren't trustworthy, they cheat, they only want you for your money, they ain't sexing you right and whatever other excuses you can find. Yet, those are the very things that you do. I mean it simply amazes me at how you *so* quickly accuse us of doing what you're doing. But guess what? *You* my dear don't even have any of those complaints, not a single one because you and I both know that it is a *fact* that I have gone out of my way to be all that you desire and more! If you ever had a complaint about me I *immediately* addressed it and corrected it. If you had any other complaints that you didn't make me aware of that went unaddressed well Si that was on you. So you don't get to use that as an excuse. So tell me why *did* you sleep with this woman? More than that why did you do whatever you did to lead her to believe that she was something more to you? Because it's clear that you've been spending quality time with this woman for her to think that. Obviously she wasn't a stick and move chick. Do you think that was fair to me or her?"

Siris paused for well over ten minutes so Aset asked him again, "What reason did you have for doing this. I made it very clear that I wasn't interested in any type of open relationship. If that's something that you're interested in than there is a very simple remedy for that. We dead this whole thing and you go ahead and do you. Besides that there are plenty of women out there who are down with sharing their man in open relationships so you would be better off with one of them. That way everybody is happy. So with that said, what I *do* know is that I am not going to waste any more of my precious time with someone who does not want the same *type* of relationship that I want. Trust me there are *plenty* of men out there who want what I want and who I could be investing my time in sharing that divine part of myself with. So I'll ask you this. Do you want the same thing that I want *and* do you want that with me? Make sure you answer that honestly. Be honest with me and more importantly be very honest with yourself."

Siris was still silent. Aset waited about 2 minutes for him to respond before interjecting saying, "Hmmmm.... Well Si I can only take your silence as a no."

With that she calmly got up to leave grabbing her purse in the same move. She was distraught and couldn't bare to look at Siris any longer. Before she could leave Siris grabbed her arm and gazed into her eyes. He knew that he had hurt Aset. He also knew that she did not deserve it and the truth was that she was right about everything. He didn't have a good reason for doing what he did. He knew that he had some maturing to do. He had trust issues with women that went back to his own relationship with his mother.

Nonetheless, he knew Aset didn't deserve to be mistreated for any of it. She was the best thing that had ever happened to him. He resolved in his mind that he was not going to lose her. He could not let her walk out of that door so he grabbed her arm to keep her from leaving. He just needed a moment to gather his thoughts and find the courage to respond. He stood staring into her eyes for about 2 minutes then he finally spoke.

"I know that what I did was wrong. I'm sorry. I apologize. I also know that I don't want to lose you because of it. I meant it when I said she meant nothing. I truly *do* want to be with you and I know you want to be with me too. You don't want to end what we've taken all this time to build anymore than I do. We both want the same thing and that's to be happy. I'm here with *you* now, no one else," Siris said as lovingly as he could.

"Hmmm. I hear you, but in this moment I just don't see you being on the same page as I am with this whole thing. Not once did you say that you too want a monogamous relationship and with me. So I am correct after all in my observation that we *don't* want the same thing. Besides that the eloquent words mean nothing if they aren't backed up by action. Love seemingly looks a lot different to me than it does you so I highly doubt I'll ever see that type of action from you. Si you are who you are and I am who I am and I have no desire to in any way change who you are to suit my fancies," Aset responded before being interrupted by Siris who was growing more agitated.

In fear that Aset was lost to him he interjected in an attempt to change her mind saying, "Baby I know you don't want to give up on and throw away all that we've built all of these years. I know you don't. You know that I love you. I know that I don't say it all the time, but I hope that I show you enough."

Pausing momentarily Aset, seemingly very serene replied, "I'll need some time to think about this. So for now I'm gonna head back to my place," Aset responded.

Maintaining the hold on her arm Siris pled with Aset with his eyes not to leave. He felt that if she walked out the door that would be the end of them and he couldn't bear the thought of that. He also wasn't convinced that she truly wanted to give up on them so easily. So he stood gazing into her eyes for about 10 more minutes.

Aset still maintained her decision to head home. She didn't want to end things with Siris, but she also didn't want to settle for less than she knew she deserved in a relationship. Besides that she wanted more and it didn't seem that Siris was ready for what she wanted. She truly did need time to think and figure out what she wanted to do.

"I truly do need some time to think. We'll speak later, but for now I just need to go," Aset said attempting to remove her arm from Si's grip.

Si would not let her go. Looking at her he was beginning to crumble inside. He couldn't believe that it had truly come to her actually leaving and it being the end of their relationship.

He knew that he couldn't force her to stay, but he didn't want to let her go. He couldn't think of anything else to say to make her stay for the moment so he went ahead and released her arm. Then the moment he let go Aset left without another word.

16

Aset was so devastated that she barely remembered the Uber ride home. She couldn't believe how one minute she was on cloud nine with Si and the next it had all just collapsed right beneath her. When she got in her apartment she sank down into the couch and began sobbing uncontrollably. During the trip home she had held it in as much as she could. So the moment she closed the door behind her the tears began streaming down her face like waterfalls. She couldn't hold them back with the strongest of her will.

Aset had given Siris all of her and in that moment she felt like such a fool for doing so. In fact, she felt like the biggest fool in history! She was in disbelief that *she* of all people had allowed herself to be played. Aset was more upset with herself than anything because for some time her intuition was telling her that Siris was seeing other women. She knew it through and through. More than that she'd seen signs of two of them. From what she gathered they both lived out of town, one in New York whom he'd occasionally fly in to see him during which time he'd wine and dine giving her even more of the royal treatment than Aset got. The other lived near Richmond, Virginia whom he'd even more often see either driving to see or having her drive to see him.

Siris was rather messy in his extracurricular dealings. Aset had seen the Richmond girl's phone number in his car one day when he asked her to help him clean it out. Besides that the Richmond girl liked to stalk him on social media in her 'indirect' attempt to make her presence known leaving telltale comments and postings on his page.

Then, in neglecting to clean up another cyber trail Siris left some other evidence on his computer knowing that Aset used his computer whenever she visited his apartment. So one day while paying a bill online for Siris Aset saw on the desktop an airline ticket and hotel receipts.

Surprisingly Aset had seen no signs of Ujana so that was a bit of a shock, which was why she was so hurt. It was one thing that he was seeing women who lived in other states, but an entirely different story that he was also seeing one locally, which likely meant more frequently. She wondered just how many other women there were.

What bothered Aset most of all was that Siris had no justification for cheating on her. She did everything for him and treated him like a king from tending to the upkeep of his home to always being there for emotional support during the trying times that he struggled through emotional breakdowns in dealing with his family drama. Most importantly, she was faithful to him and gave herself only to him. In fact, she completely opened up to him in a way that she had never opened up to anyone before. She thought that he was doing the same and seeing that she couldn't have been more wrong wounded her deeply. So she couldn't understand what reason he had for treating her that way.

Then she began thinking about and having regrets about passing up all the brothahs that would often hit on her and those who she knew from her past who had tried to get back with her whom she turned down. Many of them were very good dudes who would never have treated her so poorly. She thought about how happy she could have been in that moment if only she had chosen one of them instead.

She thought about her choices. Why did she choose Siris over all others? What a huge mistake! Aset began to feel that all that she was presently going through was all the result of her choices. Apparently she had made very poor ones and she needed desperately to understand why.

Aset must have sat on the couch sobbing for at least an hour. She cried until she didn't have anymore tears. Her guts felt like they had been ripped into a million pieces along with her heart and it seemed the pain would never subside.

Then over the course of the next couple of months it seemed that everything bad that could happen to Aset did. Her life was quickly on a downward spiral and spinning way out of control and though she tried with everything within her she was unable to engage the brakes. She'd lost her job, was one more judgement away from losing her apartment and her gallery gigs had dwindled down to nothing. In fact, with regards to her art Aset just wasn't even inspired to create anything.

She was so upset with herself for allowing Siris to get to her like this and was trying her best to turn things around for herself, but it was all to no avail. It seemed Aset had dug herself in a ditch from which she could find no escape.

Consequently, she had to ask her parents for some help in order to stay afloat, but she didn't want to burden them too much so she only asked them to help her with the bare necessities.

Meanwhile, Siris seemed to be quite happily enjoying his freedom being able to see who he wanted to see without having to sneak around to do so. He was spending a lot of time with Shauna, the woman who lived near Richmond.

To Siris Shauna was fun, easy to talk to and she was fine with how things were between them. He always felt pressured with Aset to be exclusive and Shauna didn't make him feel any of that pressure so he was able to completely be himself with her. More importantly because Shauna was okay with them not being exclusive he didn't feel so judged.

Besides all of that Shauna was a freak, not that Aset wasn't, but Shauna did more things that Aset didn't always seem so enthused about doing. Shauna was willing to do whatever, however and whenever he asked.

She was more than eager to pick up where Aset had left off and Siris felt that Shauna was a blessing for having done so.

Occasionally he called Aset, but she never accepted his calls. He knew that she'd be upset for awhile so he anticipated having to give her some time. Despite how much he was enjoying Shauna Aset was still his first love and he was determined to get her back. So he was just being patient until the time was right. In the meantime he was enjoying life. For the first time in a long time he felt like he was in high demand and for him that was his blessing.

For a while it seemed that his life was going better than ever. So he stepped things up a bit for himself, buying himself a new flat screen tv and some new furniture for his place, hanging out and partying more. Shauna had even gotten him some things for his place. For Siris, life was grand! He enjoyed being the center of attention of so many women. He felt that things were exactly as they should be.

A little over two months had passed since Aset had left Siris' house and she still had not accepted any of his calls nor had she reached out to him. She missed him terribly, but the pain in her heart would not allow her to speak to him yet. She was just as sad and disappointed at how things in their relationship had panned out as she was when she first decided to leave.

Though Aset and Siris hadn't seen one another neither of them had returned the other's apartment keys so they were not yet officially broken up. In fact, Aset was still unsure as to whether breaking up was what she even wanted to do.

Aset loved Siris deeply. He had impacted her life in a way that no man had ever done before and it was for the better. It seemed that was the very thing that was hurting her so. It was why she was so conflicted about what to do.

One evening while Aset sat on the couch contemplating things she suddenly burst into tears. It was as if the pain of it all had come flooding back into her heart again. Tears were streaming down her face like water from a faucet.

Then as if sensing her turmoil from where he was, Siris called. Aset looked at the phone blankly and did not answer. She just wasn't ready to speak to him yet. By then he had begun calling daily, but she never answered. He'd even left her a couple of voicemail messages and she could hear in his voice that he was just as sad as she was. Nonetheless, Aset maintained her silence.

That evening as Aset slowly stopped crying and sat frozen on the couch looking up to the ceiling she tried to calm her thoughts and center herself. Aset had a very strong personality and she could not let herself be defeated by the likes of Siris and his pathetic self. So she got up and walked to the bathroom.

When she got there she looked at herself in the mirror. Beginning to admire herself she looked at the structure of her doe-shaped eyes and began to appreciate their depth. She looked at her lips in awe of the perfection of their shape.

Then she took a step back and looked at the shape of her curves admiring their beauty. She looked at her voluminous curly, coily hair strands and was instantly star-struck by their strength and determination.

Lastly, she looked into the corneas of her eyes and said aloud "I love you. I love you. I love you. I love you. I love you. I love you. I love you, you beautiful, Dark goddess!"

In that moment tears began to well up in Aset's eyes again and a surge of emotion swept over her. She had the most intense feeling of adoration for herself. It was a feeling that she had never had before. Then feeling quite esteemed she slightly tilted her head to the side and gazed at herself tenderly as if she was feeling romantically attracted to herself.

She began to feel a magnetic pull from within that made her want to ravage herself as she saw staring back at her the most attractive person she'd ever before seen. It was the strangest thing because it was as if she were seeing herself as an outsider. It was almost as if she was being possessed.

Before long as if being driven by some powerful unseen force Aset went to run herself a hot bath. She also lit and then placed candles all throughout the bathroom. Next, she lit 3 sticks of frankincense cones then added some bubble bath, sea salt, essential lavender oil and a sprinkle of cinnamon to her bath water filling the tub up to the top. Lastly, she grabbed her cellphone and pushed play on her Cassandra Wilson playlist, turned the bathroom light off, undressed and slowly stepped into the tub slightly wincing as the hot water touched her skin.

Once in the tub, still feeling as though she was being possessed, Aset closed her eyes, relaxed her muscles and rested her head on the back edge of the tub. The water was so soothing and healing that it relaxed her to the point that she had, for the moment, forgotten all about the events of the day.

As she laid in the tub she entered into what was the most euphoric state of mind. It was as if she had been transported to another existence. In fact, she had. She looked around and all around her was a dim iridescent glow. It made the color of her skin take on a different color depending on what angle it was perceived from.

Then Aset was overcome by the most blissful emotional state. She felt a rapturous tingling all over her body that caused her to bend over in ecstasy. Then she heard a male voice say her name.

"Aset," he said in a deep baritone.

Aset looked around with a perplexed look on her face. The voice sounded familiar, but Aset was so far into the experience that she was having that she couldn't clearly identify who the voice belonged to. It seemed to be coming from far in the distance.

Just then she heard it again, but that time it was more gentle. She looked around for the source of the voice, but all she saw was what was the most luminous light. The light surrounded her and amidst it she felt the most intense sensation of ecstasy. It paralyzed her in bliss as she began to hear the voice calling out her name more fervently than ever. By then the elation in her intensified.

She simultaneously felt hands come out from the light that began to caress her body. The hands felt magical. They had a healing energy flowing from them that soothed and relaxed every nerve in her body. As the mysterious hands continued to explore her body Aset felt as if she was spinning. She let all resistance go and embraced the feeling of the experience.

Then just when she thought the experience couldn't get more inconceivable the unfathomable happened and absolutely blew her mind.   The male presence mounted then entered her. When it did Aset was transported to what seemed like an entirely different reality.

All around were fragrant colors.   The blacks smelled like mango, the yellows had the scent of lime, the browns smelled like peaches and there were a rainbow of other colors and scents all around. Everywhere Aset turned she saw the illumination of bright, radiant colors. It was an ocular paradise.

Meanwhile, what felt like electrical currents began to shoot through her body. Aset had never experienced anything so pleasurable in her life. She then felt a warm, electrifying, tingling sensation whiz through her causing her to yell out in ecstasy.

When she did the sound of her own voice caused her to snap out of the trip that she was on at which time she found herself back in her tub. At least she sensed that she was in her tub.   She wasn't quite sure because she still couldn't really feel her body.

It was sort of like when you wake up from a dream, but your body hasn't yet figured out the it's time to wake up. She experienced an inability to move, speak or react. It was almost as if she was in a transitional state between wakefulness and sleep.

Aset tried to focus in order to snap out of it as she was then conscious. However, she was still unable to move. Besides that she had the sensation that something was holding her down, an invisible force of some sort.

Rather than panic Aset grounded herself in an intense feeling of calm so that she could better assess what was happening. When she did she began to sense that something was very different and besides that she sensed the presence of something or someone other than herself. It was weird, but Aset felt like someone was watching her.

She went to open her eyes to see if there was someone else there but when she did she found that they would not open. Aset tried again, but still nothing. Her eyes felt like they were glued shut.

She tried to use her fingers to peel her eyes open, but that didn't work either. Then

Aset began to panic. She tried to say something, but found that she also could not speak. Then she tried again to move, but her body still would not cooperate. More than ever it was as if something was pinning her down and she felt intense pressure on her chest.

Aset tried to calm herself down. She figured that if she relaxed perhaps she would be able to snap out of it. She calmed herself down and slowed her breathing. Then she attempted again to open her eyes and raise herself up to an upright sitting position. Finally she was successful! She was able to move and open her eyes or at least it seemed like she could.

When Aset looked around it looked like her bathroom and it felt like her bathroom, yet something was different. She couldn't quite pinpoint what it was. Besides that she still sensed a presence. It was weird though because it almost felt like *she* was the presence. In fact, it felt like she was dreaming.

As she was about to get up to get out of the tub she let out a long sigh before going to lift herself up to standing position. Though when she sat up and looked in front of her she got the shock of her life! What she saw shook her to the core.

18

Aset looked up and couldn't believe her eyes. She had to blink twice to make sure that she wasn't seeing things. She thought that surely her eyes must have been playing tricks on her, but they weren't.

She took another long, hard blink and looked up again. Then she looked wide-eyed only to see that the presence that she felt was Siris! He was there with her in the tub! The whole thing took her aback and absolutely blew her mind. She had no recollection of his arrival. She wondered if he had come in while she was sort of zoned out.

Aset sat in the tub staring at Siris blankly with a million questions buzzing around in her head. For a brief moment she even felt over-exposed as if ashamed of her nakedness. Despite the fact that they'd slept together for years for some reason Aset felt like Siris had impermissibly invaded her privacy.

She wondered just how long he'd been there. How much had he seen? What was he doing there in the tub with her? Was it his voice that she heard while she was zoning out? Why was she feeling so spacey anyway?

As a thousand questions buzzed around in Aset's mind Siris sat as if oblivious to her befuddlement staring at her deeply. He was just so happy to be with Aset after such a long drawn out absence that he hadn't even noticed her awkward disposition.

Knowing that they were on the outs Siris knew that it was a risk just popping up at Aset's house and even more of a risk to use his key after she failed to answer his knocks. Nonetheless, he decided to take the chance and go see her as he couldn't bare another moment apart from her. It hurt him to the core having hurt Aset the way that he did and so he was more than happy to apologetically show her just how much he missed her.

So when he came in and found Aset in the tub and in an exceptionally good mood he figured it was as good a time as any to make up with her. Her relaxing in the tub made his timing even more felicitous so he quickly undressed and joined her.

He'd never seen Aset so open and realized that perhaps the time alone had actually done their relationship some good. He'd always heard the saying absence makes the heart grow fonder, but he never imagined that the fondness could have grown to the extent that Aset had displayed it.

The moment he got into the tub it was as if Aset was an ocean that engulfed him. Instantly he was swept away into what seemed a tidal wave of affection. It was like the tidal wave that didn't end because Aset seemed to climax for at least half an hour. In the meantime, she gave him sensations that he could never have conceptualized. Aset had taken him to heaven. Yet, when the bliss of their love-making ended and Aset looked around in befuddlement suddenly the coldness of Aset's negative disposition caused Siris to feel as if he had been violently expelled from a hurricane.

Though they hadn't yet exchanged words once Siris came out of the daze of their lovemaking he sensed a piercingly abrupt awkwardness develop between them. At first Siris thought that it was the awkwardness that always lingers during the early phases of the make-up period after a fight. However, he realized that was not the case as he sensed that Aset was not in the least bit happy about his being there.

So he figured perhaps he just needed to give her time to process everything for a minute. He realized that his popping up may have caught her off guard and that since they had both snapped out of the whirlwind of their lovemaking perhaps it was all hitting her all at once. So he figured that he should wait to speak until he felt the time was right. Then about 5 minutes later he finally spoke.

"So I missed you." Siris said with some hesitation and an inkling of embarrassment for having popped up on her the way that he had.

As they both sat naked in the tub facing one another with Aset's legs resting on the top of Siris he gently grabbed ahold of her hands and looked into her eyes as he spoke to her. As Aset began to come back into her own wits she began to feel the coolness of the water as she had been in the tub for quite awhile and thus the warmth had disappeared.

She was still very confused about things, particularly how Siris got there and the reason for his seemingly calm demeanor. She looked around and was somewhat relieved that she was at least in the comfort of her own home because despite what her eyes showed her it felt as though she was somewhere else. She could still smell the fragrance of the incense. The soft glow of the candles made her relax a bit, but the feeling of Siris' touch made her feel an uneasiness. Aset had no idea what was going on.

Though when she looked around everything seemed familiar. However, it didn't *feel* that way. It felt as if part of her was somewhere else.

Momentarily, it all reminded Aset of past life visions. It was a vision where she as the Dark Goddess was an Earth. It was a vision that she had experienced as a painful memory, one that was her present as much as it was her past.

As the vision went one day while enjoying the bliss of her own femininity in darkness the Dark Goddess began to feel the sensation of being shaken up and yanked out of herself. She resisted with all of her being, but it was to no avail because a force more intense than her own seemed to overtake her. It overtook her to the point that it shifted the entire focus of her energy forcing it to physically manifest in an inverted form.

Before she could even process what was happening she realized that she had manifested as an Earth. This caused her to feel both outraged and perplexed because

Earth was a form that had previously only been manifested by a masculine nature. So having been forced into a form contrary to her current energetic focus was likened to a woman being forced to possess a man's body.

Nothing felt right. It threw the entire cosmos off balance, which was in violation of the divine order of things. Consequently, chaos erupted throughout the entire cosmos!

The Dark Goddess had no idea who had caused such a disruption, but she was determined to not only find out *who* had done it, but *why*?

The Dark Goddess focused to calm herself so that she could get a better sense of exactly what was going on. As she focused, she began to sense that there was a presence lurking about. Despite its attempt to mask its intentions it felt mischievous, menacing and cunning and the Dark Goddess knew that she needed to stay on guard. The presence did not give off a very respectful quality. In fact, it seemed to lack any respect for who she was.

The Dark Goddess continued to read the energy of the presence as she attempted to come up with a strategy to guard herself. As she focused in on it she concluded that the presence did in fact pose a threat and that soon it would strike out against her.

For some reason the Dark Goddess sensed that the presence was feeling dissatisfied. She thought that perhaps the dissatisfaction was the reason why it acted out by disrupting things the way that it had. She still didn't have an answer to the bigger question, which was WHY?

All throughout the cosmos was blissful. There was nothing to be dissatisfied about. The Dark Goddess was happily coexisting with her illuminated companion as they had finally reached a point of perfect balance. This is what made it all the more perplexing as to why any form could experience dissatisfaction to the point of so drastically disrupting things.

The cosmos had its cycles of highs and lows as was the universal law. However, the disturbance that had just been caused had dealt a devastating blow to all in existence and was far more than a normal cycle of highs and lows. It was like someone had set off a nuclear bomb in the middle of an oasis. It made no sense.

In the balanced universe Earth was animated by a masculine form as the body while the sky was animated by a feminine form as the mind. Together they were the perfect pair as her calm, introspective passivity was the perfect complement to his constant flow of activity as Earth had always been one of the most sprightly and life-giving planetary forms. She was his heaven in an ever-changing, volatile world and he was the magnetic, gravitational pull that kept her grounded, giving her a sense of order in her chaotic darkness.

As a result of the recent imbalance the heavens were no more. Instead, there was left only a constant carnation of one hellish reality after another, as an abyss of what seemed like an eternity of suffering. Particularly for the Dark Goddess, occupying a form so contrary to her nature and her purpose was a most hellish experience. It was the horrific dream that she wanted to end.

The more she thought about it the more she wanted to see truth revealed and for the one behind the damnation of her heaven to make itself known. Just then the Dark Goddess saw it. She saw the illumination of his light. It shown like an inferno and it was then that she realized that she was trapped in a perpetual cycle of hell on Earth.

The Dark Goddess cried out, but there was no one to hear her. Feeling empowered and revelling in the display of his might he arrogantly revealed himself to her catching her off guard. Then without giving her a chance to defend, like a predator he pounced. Then again and again he invaded her in this way, having his way with her in every manner that he desired. Each time he finished he'd tell her how good she was and how the feeling of her was something he wanted again and again and again as it made him rise.

Seeing who he was devastated the Dark Goddess more than the violence against her.

For her it was the most duplicitous of betrayals. It was a broken trust that could never be repaired.

Thinking back on the vision Aset suddenly felt the same way. Upon seeing that the presence that she was sensing was Siris Aset felt that his being there was a violation of her divine space. She felt that Siris had permanently broken her trust and therefore had no right to forcefully interject himself into her space. So contrary to what Siris expected, happy to see him Aset was not.

19

Finally coming back to her senses Aset looked deeply into Siris' eyes. As she looked into his eyes she still had the feeling that somehow she wasn't where she appeared to be. It was like she was watching herself in a movie. She thought to herself that perhaps she was dreaming so she decided to test the theory by speaking to Siris to see if he would respond.

"Hmmph. How did you get here? I didn't let you in? As a matter of fact, I didn't hear you come in," Aset inquired with unexpected calm anxious to hear a response so that she knew that she was alive and it was all really happening.

Aset needed some confirmation that she wasn't losing her mind and she somehow knew that Si's response would confirm it for her.

"I know I shouldn't have, but I let myself in. I knocked a few times and when you didn't answer I thought that you may have been asleep or in the shower so I decided to use my key. I tried calling too, but you haven't been taking my calls so I had no choice but to come on over," Siris said with a hint of humiliation.

Staring at him blankly and feeling no emotion Aset was too preoccupied with finding an explanation for the apparent out-of-body-experience that she was having to even begin to take an interest in addressing the unresolved issues between she and Siris.

Hearing Siris respond directly to her question Aset concluded that she wasn't dreaming and therefore ruled that out. Yet she still had no other explanation, only a feeling. It felt as if she had separated from herself and was capturing a remote view of what was going on around her body. It was the most uncanny experience.

Interrupting her thoughts in an attempt to shift the mood Siris blurted out, "Well that was *some* welcome you just gave me there! I see you missed me just as much as I missed you."

The moment Siris spoke Aset got the most eerily familiar feeling and she was suddenly overcome with dread. It was like dèjá vu.

Something about Siris reminded her of the God in her vision. It was the part about her being transformed into an Earth. Aset suddenly became angry because the last part of what she remembered was that the Dark Goddess' illuminated love, Amaz was the mysterious perpetrator who had transformed her. When she learned of his identity she was furious! Aset was suddenly feeling the same emotions as she was in her vision.

So when Siris spoke using the words that he had in the tone that he had spoken in it instantly took Aset back to Amaz, who was the Dark Goddess' love from a past life. There was something about Siris' choice of words that triggered this memory and it wasn't a pleasant one.

Aset was beginning to feel skeptical of Siris. She began questioning who he really was and what his true intentions were. The events that had occurred were freaking her out and she was having trouble identifying just what was real and what wasn't anymore.

Aset sat for several moments silently looking at Siris. Physically he looked the same, but there was something very different about him now that she could see him with her more remote eyes.

She got a more crafty, sly impression of him than she had noticed before. She couldn't believe how she missed seeing that about him before. It wasn't a new characteristic that had just shown up. It had been there all along. It was the same fraudulence that she somehow remembered from her vision and that was giving her a feeling of dèjá vu.

As she was deep in thought about what was happening something else happened that made things even stranger. She looked around and for a brief moment everything went dark. It was like a momentary blackout or a brief period of blindness so to speak.

It wasn't really blindness though because she still felt as though she could see, but just in a different way. It was as if she could see things as feelings. This lasted for at least a minute if time could even be applied.

During that time Aset felt a familiar sense of formlessness. It seemed as though she was somehow disappearing. Then in what seemed like the blink of an eye she was back, at least back in the sense that things came back into focus for her and was no longer dark.

More confused than ever Aset looked deeper into Siris' eyes to see if she'd find any answers there. Several minutes had passed by and she just sat there staring at him. It seemed to make Siris very uncomfortable so he nervously looked away feeling very confused by what was happening.

However, just when Aset was finally about to say something to Siris there was a knock at the door. From the sound of it the person knocking had a sense of urgency.

Aset looked at Siris perplexed as if she had no idea who could be at the door. The person knocked again so Siris jumped up, quickly got dressed to go see who was at the door leaving Aset some extra time to get some clothes on. When he promptly made his way to the door Siris reached for the doorknob and looked through the peephole and saw that it was Aset's friend, Tisha.

He turned to yell back to Aset and said, "It's Tisha," as he unlocked the door to let her in.

"Hey Tisha! How are you? Come on in. Aset will be right out," Siris greeted as Tisha walked in slowly having not expected Siris to be the one to answer the door.

It was around 10 o'clock at night and Tisha never came over that late. However, Siris didn't usually answer the door whenever she did stop by.

Siris made small talk with Tisha as they both headed for the livingroom to give Aset a moment to get herself together.

"So how have you been Tisha? I haven't seen you in a while. How is the family?" Siris said warmly.

"Hi Siris. It's good seeing you. The family is fine," Tisha responded looking around for signs of her having possibly disturbed Siris and Aset popping up so late.

Meanwhile, hearing Tisha's voice Aset struggled in the bathroom trying to quickly get herself together. The sensation of being out of her body made it very difficult to *control* her movements. It felt like she was one person trying to control the body of another.

In another sense it was like her mind was separated from her body and her mind was having the most difficult time getting her body to do what she ordered it to do. Nonetheless, Aset eventually got a handle on it and soon she was able to get some clothes on and walk herself to the living room.

However, the more Aset got a handle on, the more strange things popped up which she wasn't so quickly able to control. When she saw Tisha despite all of her efforts, she had the most difficult time emoting. She tried to make her mouth form a smile, but it would not obey. So she hugged Tisha with what unfortunately came off as a very cold reception.

"Hi Tisha, what brings you here this time of night?" Aset greeted without a hint of emotion.

Looking at Siris as if hinting that she wanted some privacy Tisha responded, "Oh just out for a breather."

Siris got the hint and headed towards Aset's bedroom to give them some privacy. Meanwhile, Aset joined Tisha on the couch to talk. Tisha looked anxious so Aset decided to get to the point to find out what was going on.

However, before she could ask Tisha blurted out, "Girl sorry to interrupt your evening, but I needed an alibi."

Ordinarily Tisha's statement would have annoyed Aset. Though strangely enough with all that was going on Aset felt a sense of detachment from her friend's problems. However, in an effort to appear as sane as possible Aset struggled to find the appropriate human responses so as to come off halfway normal.

So doing the best that she could trying to somehow survive the visit as she mustered up some resemblance of perplexity Aset asked, "What? Why do you need an alibi?"

"Girl I needed to get out of that house. I just couldn't take it anymore. I'm tired of sacrificing and not having anything left for me. I needed some damn 'me' time. So I left Eric there with the kids and as for me…" Tisha said slyly before smiling and pausing.

"What is it Tish? What are you up to?" Aset asked still struggling to show signs of genuine interest.

Tisha smiled and said proudly, "I have a date!"

"What!?!!!!" Aset exclaimed still trying to exert some mastery over her voice volume and expression.

"Yep. I'm going out with Brian. He's meeting me at an Italian restaurant in Arlington in a few minutes. I stopped by here so that I can say, with a clear conscious, that I was with you."

Still feeling no emotion about what Tisha had said Aset tried to find the right words in response to appear as her normal overbearing self, whatever that was anymore.

"Hmmm is that so? Well do you girl, but I already told you how I feel about your whole sneaking around with Brian fling. I hope you know what you're doing and that this doesn't blow up in your face," Aset calmly replied finally getting back into the flow of things.

"Girl I got this. Anyway I have to get going. I want to be fashionably late, but I don't want Brian to think that I stood him up so I have to head out. I'll call you tomorrow to tell you how it goes," Tisha said damn near bolting out of the door excitedly.

"Ok girl. Talk to you later!" Aset yelled out after Tisha.

As Aset closed the door behind Tisha she suddenly had the most prophetic inkling. It gave her some clarity about what was going on with her.

However, before she could get too deep in thought about it having heard Aset let Tisha out Siris figured it was okay to come out of the room. So taking each step gingerly he came tiptoeing out of the room to join Aset who he saw was sitting on the couch apparently deep in thought.

"Hey baby. So how was Tisha? Everything alright? Haven't known her to come by so late," Siris inquired trying to lighten the air between them that had despite his efforts quickly returned to a tense state.

"Yeah she's fine. She was just hanging out for the evening for some grown up time," Aset answered trying to be discreet.

"Oh, did she want the two of you to hang out? You could have gone. I would have been okay with it," Siris said.

"Oh no it's fine. I wouldn't have gone anyway. That was too late notice. She went out with another friend and was stopping by here on the way to blow some time because she was early," Aset said.

One thing that Aset wasn't was a snitch in or out of her body. She was not a friend to betray anyone's trust so she kept to herself what was going on with Tisha. Besides that she and Si no longer shared so intimate a relationship where she was willing to share anything personal with him.

Changing the subject Siris said, "So anyway back to us. Where did *we* leave off?"

Siris was very anxious to see where Aset's head was with regards to their relationship. He knew that one sexual encounter, no matter how mind-blowing, was going to be the catalyst that got their relationship back on track. He also knew that Aset was a very introverted person who tended to keep her thoughts to herself. So finding out exactly what was in her head would be no easy feat. She was never as transparent as she let on.

Nonetheless, as he gazed into her eyes he longed to see that the deeply penetrative stare that he saw was focused on him. Though as he saw the blankness in her stare he knew that wasn't the case and worried that it would never again be.

20

Without responding Aset calmly got up and went to bed. She suddenly needed to sleep. Siris sat dumbfounded. He didn't know what to think. It was as if Aset could have cared less about him and almost seemed to forget that he was even there. He sat on the couch for the next few hours until he too drifted off to sleep.

Though Aset had gone to bed and her body lay asleep her mind was wide awake and seemingly still very separate from her body. Aset still had lots of questions about what was going on and so she spent most of the night trying to sort things out. Her mind was racing and no matter what she did she couldn't put it to rest so she also spent some time practicing different ways to control her body and emotions. It did a lot of good because by morning she had mastered both quite well and though Aset had stayed up the entire night strangely enough she didn't feel at all tired.

The next morning Siris slept on the couch until about 11 o'clock. It was Aset's loudly ringing cell phone, which had been left sitting on the loveseat that woke him up.

Aset came running out of her bedroom to get her phone. It was Tisha, but Aset was not yet ready to talk so she chose to ignore the call and made a mental note to call back later. Tisha was no doubt calling to tell Aset about the details of her steamy date with Brian and Aset didn't want to discuss it in front of Siris.

Looking over at her Siris greeted, "Good morning sleepyhead. I was wondering when you'd wake up. I woke up earlier then went back to sleep after seeing that you were still sleeping so soundly. I guess that all nighter got the best of you."

"Yeah I guess it did," Aset answered as if she knew what Siris was talking about. Meanwhile, her mind was in knots. As far as she knew she had been up all night while Siris slept. She had no recollection of them having sex.

Was her body acting on it's own? Had she blacked out again? If it wasn't a dream what *was* it? Before she could get too far into dissecting the whole thing in her head again Siris interrupted her thoughts.

"So tell me how do you feel about everything, everything that happened yesterday and how it changes everything between us? I guess you *could* say it puts us on an entirely different track," Siris said looking at Aset intensely.

"Well I'm not really sure. Still processing things," Aset said in a contemplative tone.

With a look of disappointment Siris nodded his head in the affirmative to signify that he understood Aset's position. He knew that things would take some time to get back to normal and was prepared to give Aset the time she needed.

Just then Aset's phone rang interrupting their conversation yet again. It was Tisha again. That time her phone was in plain view and because Aset figured Siris had seen that it was Tisha as she noticed him glancing at it she picked the phone up.

"You can go ahead. I'm going to get me a drink. Did you want one too?" Siris asked as he got up to head to the kitchen.

"No I'm fine," Aset answered while simultaneously hitting the answer button on her phone.

Once she saw that Siris was out of the room she answered the phone saying, "Hey girl! What's going on? Sorry I missed your call earlier."

"Giiiiiiiirrrrrlllllll what ain't going on? I'll give you the good stuff first. So last night with Brian….. absolutely amazing! He still lights me up with just a glance. I mean girl his kindness, his generosity, making me feel like a queen, taking the time to actually listen to me rather than being so self-absorbed in his own stuff just made me fall in love with him all over again. In fact that's why I'm going out to lunch with him on Tuesday. Now before you say it I know you're gonna say slow down and not to jeopardize what I have with Eric over this, but I swear to you that I've thought a lot about what I'm doing. Eric and I were good while we lasted, but girl that ship has sailed and last night was confirmation of that for me. I know it was. Last night was the first time in a long time that I actually enjoyed myself. I actually felt like someone appreciated me for me and understood me," Tisha rambled while bubbling over with excitement on the other end of the phone.

Exhaling deeply before responding, still emotionless, Aset replied, "Tisha I hear you and I even understand where you are with this, but I have to say that I'm sure you know relationships are riddled with ups and downs and sometimes during the course of your relationship there can appear to be more downs than ups. Truthfully it's all about perception and where you are in the scheme of things. Right now you're feeling disappointment and rejection and you're acting out as a result."

Interrupting Tisha said, "Yeah Aset, I already know where you're going with this and I don't want to hear it. You're not going to sit here and tell me that I'm supposed to settle for what I'm getting out of my marriage. That I'm supposed to be doing all of this myself. I didn't have these kids by myself so I shouldn't be the only one tending to their needs while he just comes home and sits on his ass everyday or is just here, there, everywhere, coming and going as he damn well pleases while I'm stuck with the kids. I'm sick of that shit and there are fathers, husbands, boyfriends out here who *do* help with the kids and *aren't* living in the cave man era beating their chest talking about 'woman do as I say!"

"That's not what I'm saying Tisha. What I'm saying is that what you're expecting from Eric, or anyone for that matter, is not reasonable. You're expecting him to be responsible for how you feel and it's impossible for anyone to control how *you* feel or you them," Aset responded.

Tisha sighed deeply on the other end of the phone indicating frustration by what Aset was saying.

"Just hear me out," Aset said acknowledging Tisha's vexation, "If in your relationship you are feeling under-appreciated, undesirable, insignificant and all of these things it is you who are projecting that into your own reality. You grumble about what you don't get from your relationships with your husband, your children, your co-workers and whoever else. Yet you never take the time to enjoy what they all provide for you that is desirable. So what you get back is a perfect match to what you give in these relationships. You just can't see that because right now you can only see things from the perspective of a victim. So you see everything as some mass conspiracy to make your life miserable. You're making you miserable by focusing so much on the things that make you miserable. You feel happy with

Brian for the moment because it's new and that's what you're choosing to focus on. Well that's a prime example of how you are in control of your reality. If you choose to focus on those things that make you happy then you see the manifestation of that in your life. You could just as easily do the same where you stand right now in your current family and enjoy a whole new reality."

On the other end of the phone Tisha wondered exactly *who* she was talking to? It sounded nothing like her friend. She was calling to share some exciting news about her date and yet she was getting berated by her so-called best friend. Who *was* she talking to? It felt more like she was on the line with a therapist than her best friend and that began to really piss Tisha off.

So abruptly interrupting Aset Tisha said, "But it's more than that. Truth be told Eric is not even my type. Brian was always more my type. He's probably who I should have married to begin with. I always saw myself with an educated, more executive corporate type man.

He's close to his mama and you know what they say about how men treat their mama. You know the issues Eric has with his mama. I mean the way he talks to her girl shows me that he just doesn't respect women and he never will. He doesn't appreciate me and most of all I don't feel like he even knows how to love me," Tisha defended.

Hearing the last sentence of what Tisha had just said seemed to have rung louder than all the others and so Aset promptly asked, "Girl what did you just say? Did you do what I think you did last night?"

"Ha! A good girl never tells! But like I said, last night was absolutely amazing," Tisha screeched.

Seeing that Tisha was not yet ready to fully receive what she was communicating Aset decided to end the conversation. She knew that Tisha was going to do what she wanted to do. Her mind was already made up and nothing that Aset said was going to make a difference. Besides that Aset wanted to get back to her own issues. She wanted to get back to figuring out what happened with her last night and what Si was talking about. So she decided to wrap up her conversation with Tisha seeing that it wasn't going anywhere anyway.

At the same time in that instance Aset was overcome by a rush of energy. It was the most invigorating feeling that she had ever experienced. It was as if a shower of pure, positive energy had just rained down on her and she felt most refreshed.

Abruptly bringing the conversation to a close so she could fully absorb that good feeling Aset said "Well girl I know that you're gonna take care and do what's best for you, but I hope that you consider what I've said. We can chat more about it later if you want. I have to go for now though because Si is still here and I'm being rather rude."

"Oh girl go ahead. I'm so sorry for tying up you all this time. Tell him my apologies. We'll chat later girl! Peace!" Tisha said before hanging up.

Aset knew that Tisha was upset with her for speaking to her in such a tone, but suddenly, almost instantaneously, Aset had no regrets, no guilt about it and the most euphoric, liberating sense of detachment from the whole thing.

21

The next several days were a bit of a blur. Life as Aset knew it had forever changed. She had not slept since the night of the incident in the tub, at least she had not slept mentally. It seemed that her body went on to have a life of its own where it did as it had always routinely done eating, drinking, sleeping and carrying out all of its other bodily functions. It was like she was a shell of herself. Her body just went through its daily motions almost like a robot.

Later Aset learned that hers was not an isolated case. There were several other Carbo women describing similar incidents including her twin sister, Bast. They all described a feeling of not quite being themselves. Some even described it as being seemingly immaterial. It was abuzz all throughout the community.

Meanwhile, Aset's mind was experiencing an entirely different reality. Her mind was more vibrant than ever. She discovered that it had powers way beyond her wildest imagination. It had become the mind that didn't sleep. While her body slept it seemed her mind expanded. As it did Aset transported herself to all the places she always dreamt of going. She travelled across time, across realities and visited with other beings. She was even able to intuit things and make connections between things. During the course of all of this Aset intuitively sensed more about what was happening to her and many other Carbo women.

It happened one night while her body rested that her mind put it all together. Aset could see the unfolding of it as clear as day, in a vision.

The vision revealed to her that they were very ancient Goddesses who had been imprisoned as Earths by Amaz. Lifetime after lifetime Amaz had forcefully extracted Goddesses one by one from their Source transforming them into Earths then forcing them to submit to his carnal desires. He begrudgingly degraded them treating them as his sex slaves and in other cases conning them with his trickery to do as he pleased.

The most beautiful ones who would often also be the most resistant he lied to and told them that they were the love for whom he'd searched the universe to find. The strongest and most powerful of them he used whatever chicanery it took to get them to let down their guard so that he could have his way with them. He was like a wild, parent-less child with no boundaries or self-control and there weren't enough Goddesses in the universe to ever quench his gluttonous appetite. His juvenile immaturity so amplified his lust such that he eventually forbid the Earths to reveal but the slightest hint of their flesh. So he covered them all three quarters of the way in water.

Amaz was a savage brute in his dealings with the Goddesses, which was not the trait of any of the other Gods. He was the tyrant of the universe and for many lifetimes many attempted to take him down without success. For whenever they would come for Amaz, being the coward that he was, he would hide in the womb of one of his Earths.

However, recently the Goddesses had somehow devised a way to mentally extract themselves from the prison that was then their human bodies.

Amaz was always paranoid about the Goddesses escaping from their Earthly forms so he embodied them into human flesh as women as an insurance policy and to quell his insecurities. Additionally, so that he could continue to partake in his carnal desires he would from time to time carnate himself as human flesh as well. Immediately he discovered that human form was one of his favorite ways to enjoy his lustful pleasures. In human form he could better control the Goddesses minds and he could more easily physically subdue them as in his human form he had the advantage of brute strength. As man, Amaz ruled the Earths and as such he more adeptly ruled the Goddesses.

Eventually, he convinced them that they were of no divine origin and were instead merely his companions and instruments of pleasure. He used his cunning and trickery to cause them to completely forget who they were. Amaz's power of enchantment was irreproachable. He was so adept at this talent that he could convince even the brightest of them to renounce her very being and see it as a sin.

Forgotten were the Goddesses who were once the heavens, the wombs from which all of creation sprung. They were the aspect of Source that inspired thought. Their transcendent beauty adorned the heavens making it bliss. They were the Gods' co-creators. They were the half of God that made him whole. Yet, all of this Amaz forced the

Goddesses to alienate, which in turn forced them to become alien to even themselves.

However, somewhere along the way something happened. Something happened that changed everything and somehow turned the tables. It happened the day, the hour, the moment that Aset was in the tub.

Perhaps it was an oversight on Amaz's part. Perhaps his guard was down. Perhaps there was a glitch in his matrix. Whatever it was, Goddesses all over the planet and throughout many other worlds began to free themselves from their bodies, at least mentally. When they did this it changed the nature of everything.

The tides had changed and it was in favor of the Goddesses. For all over the universe Goddesses were remembering who they were. Slowly they were rediscovering their power. Most importantly they were overcoming their pain....

As Aset continued to intuit what all started to blend together as the past, present and future she wondered what the fate of she and the rest of the Carbo women was. As much as life as they knew it still seemed normal, what she was intuiting was far from normal. There was dissatisfaction among the women and one way or another Aset knew that soon it all had to play itself out.

She wondered if that was already happening by way of so many Carbo women acting on impulses to leave their families. Perhaps that was just the beginning. Perhaps it meant that *everything* was about to change and that the Carbo woman that used to be was no more.

22

A week later Aset's inkling would be confirmed when she went to the bookstore as was her habit. When she got there things were not at all what she expected. It seemed that everywhere she turned there was a Carbo couple either arguing or lustfully all over each other and violently so. In fact, Aset thought that at any moment they may all just spontaneously combust.

The fighting couples were on the verge of coming to blows while the hot and bothered couples acted like they were about to start an orgy right in the middle of the street at any minute. Perplexed as to what was happening Aset decided to explore further.

When she did, Aset unexpectedly saw a familiar face. She couldn't believe her eyes so she had to do a double take. When she looked again she confirmed that her eyes were in fact not deceiving her. It was Tisha, but what was unexpected was that Tisha was with Brian and she was all over him! Though still emotionless, Aset did not expect to see that Tisha was so bold as to be parading around town with Brian, who was *not* her husband.

Just then, Tisha had spotted Aset and instantly ran up to her smiling ear to ear and bubbling over with excitement hand in hand with Brian. Almost skipping and gleeful as ever Tisha shrieked loudly then broke her hand away from Brian's and ran over to greet Aset.

"Hey you! What a surprise seeing you out here in the suburbs. What are you doing here? Catching a movie? That's where we're about to go," Tisha exclaimed giving Aset a hug, while gazing at Brian seductively.

Before answering Aset glanced over at Brian, then turned to Tisha waiting for an introduction. Seeing Aset glance over at Brian reminded Tisha that she had not formally introduced him.

"Oh I'm so rude sometimes. Brian this is my best friend Aset who you may remember from Blair. She went to high school with us," Tisha said grabbing Brian's hand again and pointing to Aset.

With a bright smile Brian instantly went to extend his hand to Aset to greet her, "Hey Aset, I think you do look rather familiar. Nice to meet you."

Aset's reception, though skeptical was warm as she returned the handshake.

Sensing the awkwardness and seeing the confused look written all over Aset's face Tisha decided to cut the introduction short saying, "Well I don't want to be late to this movie or hold you up so we're gonna get moving. It was good seeing you girl. Enjoy your evening out and I'll chat with you later!"

Then in an instant before Aset could even render a farewell pleasantry Tisha and Brian had disappeared. Then in the next moment it seemed that everything began to speed up so fast that Aset didn't have time to process it.

Suddenly everything around Aset began to happen at hypersonic speeds. It was so much so that she began to wonder if she was the one causing things to speed up. The more her thoughts went into overdrive so did the events around her. One thought birthed another and another, which seemed to birth 100 others until it seemed a multitude of thoughts in the form of Carbo people swarmed around Aset like a tornado.

Feeling the power within her surge Aset, who was then the eye of the storm that had formed around her, calmly closed her physical eyes and inhaled deeply. Though when she closed her physical eyes it seemed a set of, what felt like electric eyes opened in their place.

With that her primary senses heightened making her physical senses secondary. Instantly Aset could sense the emotional feelings of everyone around her as thoughtforms. She could sense their true and deepest desires. She could even see thru beyond their physical forms. They become light beings until the light around her became near blinding.

Feeling the need to restore some balance and to calm the storm around her Aset then closed all of her eyes. When she did she experienced what was like a penetrating darkness, which appeared as some sort of vortex like a black hole. In this black hole Aset felt the most euphoric feeling of satisfaction. It was as if in this vortex all that she ever desired existed and made Aset feel an instance of happiness and love that she had never before experienced. She never wanted to leave. However, the more she longed to stay the stronger a force around her became that pulled at her yanking her out.

Then for a brief moment all around her became stillness, immediately followed by a gang of the light beings overpowering Aset as she had not yet mastered her own stillness. The lightning beings violently yanked Aset out of the dark vortex causing Aset to feel an agonizing pain. Unable to control herself Aset screamed out in pain. Yet to the external world the scream was silent because in reality Aset was experiencing the whole thing in her mind.

Thus, instead of coming out as a scream Aset's scream was a feeling of implosion. It was as if her entire being imploded and the pain felt was even more torturous than the pain Aset felt after being yanked out of the dark vortex. She began to feel that something was familiar about what she was experiencing. It felt much like the time that she was separated from herself as the Dark Goddess and made into an earth.

However, before Aset could put the pieces together to understand what was happening advancing toward her were what appeared to be lightning spears that in truth were the deepest of her hellish thoughtforms who were then collectively waging the most violent of attacks. Overcome by the worst of all that she'd ever contemplated Aset continued to implode as the lightning spears struck her from all angles.

With each piercing of a lightning spear Aset experienced a most hellish pain that penetrated every aspect of her being.

Seemingly they took on the faces of all of those that she had at one point in time perceived as an enemy from family members and close friends to mere passersby on the street. This all caused her head to ache in ways that her mind could have never before conceived. However, unbeknownst to Aset the worst was still yet to come.

Struggling to maintain herself with all of her will Aset tried again to absorb all that was around her into her darkness. Yet again she was unsuccessful as her dominance was merely transitory.

Somehow she had to figure a way to block them all out to give herself a chance to focus inward long enough to maintain control. However, each time she attempted to do so it seemed another multitude of lightning spears more lethal than the last would appear and subdue her efforts.

The more momentum they gained the stronger they became and the weaker Aset became. She began feeling light-headed as if she would mentally faint, if that were at all possible. Yet the uncontrollable state that Aset found herself in seemed quite riddled with all sorts of unanticipated and unexpected possibilities so she was ready for just about anything.

Then as if it were the next logical thing that could happen in a script in a movie the worst of her lightning spear-headed thoughtforms appeared..... as Siris.

23

Towering over her the light emanating from Siris was near blinding and Aset had to look away just to maintain her composure. She had to put her hand up as if shielding her eyes from the sun, which was odd to onlookers because it was well after sunset.

"Hey baby is everything alright. You look like you've been through hell. What happened?" Siris said looking concerned.

Struggling to regain her composure and try to understand what was going on Aset slowly responded saying, "I just suddenly have a really bad headache."

She was trying to understand how Siris got there and why. She only remembered coming to the bookstore by herself. More than that she couldn't for the life of her understand why he appeared to her as such a blinding light. The only way that she could converse with him was by looking down. The light emanating from Siris was so blinding that Aset could barely make out that it was even Siris. She was really only able to identify him on the basis of the familiarity of his presence.

"Oh I'm sorry baby. I could have just met you at your place. You didn't have to meet me up here if you weren't feeling well. Do you need for me to go and get you something for your headache? There's a grocery store on the other side of the parking lot," Siris inquired.

"No you don't have to do that. I have something. I think I just need to head home. We'll have to postpone this if you don't mind," Aset replied convincingly.

Still trying to regain some understanding of all that was happening to her Aset was feeling unusually anxious and wanted nothing more than to get to her car. Standing there talking to Siris while still seeing lightning spears all around Aset was feeling very exposed and felt that getting to her car would help her feel more secure.

Seeing her discomfort Siris offered, "Sure. Let's head back. I'll walk you to your car then we can meet up at your place so you can get some rest."

Aset agreed and Siris walked her to her car. Once she got into her car Aset felt like she had finally found shelter from a tornado. For some reason her car felt like a protective force field that shielded her from danger. She sat, closed her eyes and breathed deeply for a moment just to get herself back in sync with what she remembered as her reality. It took a moment but soon she was back to the closest resemblance of normal that she could recall.

She drove back home and the entire way as she pondered all that had transpired she felt like she was struggling to solve a riddle. She thought about seeing Tisha and how weird that encounter was. Then she recalled how quickly things took a turn for the worst and wondered what it all meant.

It was as if her thoughts were attacking her. It seemed one paralyzing thought multiplied into millions and within an instant. Before long they gained momentum and launched attacks from which Aset could not find shelter.

Finally, after what seemed like forever Aset arrived at her apartment to find that Siris had beat her there. He was waiting for her outside as she pulled up looking very worried.

As she pulled into a parking space Siris walked up to meet her at the car and to open her door.

"You finally made it hunh. I was wondering what was taking you so long and if you were okay," Siris said as he closed Aset's car door behind her.

"I'm fine. I was just taking my time I guess," Aset said still squinting at the sight of Siris.

The light emanating from him wasn't as blinding as it was earlier, but it was still difficult for Aset to absorb. She wondered how she would endure the remainder of his visit especially once they got inside. She decided that looking at him from her peripheral would be best.

Once they made it into the apartment Aset went straight to her room to prepare herself for a much needed shower while Siris sat in the living room watching tv. As the water ran down her body so did the anxiety from the day's events. Aset slowly began to calm down and soon returned to her more peaceful disposition. She no longer saw the lightning spears as her thoughts too began to take on a more peaceable quality.

As she turned off the shower and dried herself Aset felt refreshed. She stepped onto the mat just outside of her tub then walked over to the mirror and looked at her reflection in the eye. As she did she noticed a sort of dark glow about her. It was much like the iridescent glow of a black light bulb. She hadn't noticed it before, but in that moment it stood out to her as prominently as the bright light emanating from Siris.

She looked at her glow and smiled slyly unable to mask even from herself her sense of pride in it. Leaving out of the bathroom to return to her room to slip on some comfortable lounging clothes Aset returned to her normal state. Her home felt like a much needed shelter and she was so glad to be back in it.

Siris had found a football game on tv and was engrossed in the game so that he hadn't noticed how long Aset had been absent from the room. She was relieved that he'd found something to occupy his mind other than her and welcomed the break from being the center focus of his attention.

They spent the remainder of the evening without much conversation and later that night Siris got a call from Chris and decided to go out. It was a welcomed break from him that Aset needed so she took advantage of the night alone to continue getting herself back on track.

Her out-of-body sensation was the same. However, there seemed to be a more dark quality about her. It was dark in a sinister sort of way and Aset had taken a liking to it.

Something about the attack that Aset had endured had drawn something else out of her. It seemed to come from somewhere in the depths of her and it was intoxicating.

Later that night as Aset lay in the bed the phone rang. Aset looked at the clock and it was 3:15am so she knew who it was before she even looked at the phone.

"You asleep?" Siris said on the other end.

"Does it matter now?" Aset responded blankly.

"I guess not. Just getting in my car and was thinking about coming back by there. You want me to come?" Siris queried.

Aset took a long pause before responding. She was quite enjoying her time alone. It seemed she spent more time with Siris than she did herself and she wasn't sure that she was ready to end the visit so abruptly.

Annoyed at her hesitation Siris said, "Well I guess that means no. I'll just head home then and talk to you tomorrow."

Before Aset could reply Siris had hung up the phone annoyed. Aset smiled to herself relieved to have dodged what would have been an unwelcome visit. She felt no guilt about having offended Siris. She needed time by herself to get back intuned with who she was and so she joyously used the time to do just that.

24

The next morning Aset rose from her bed with a renewed sense of being. She seemed to bask in the wonder of it all for at least an hour before finally getting out of the bed. It was a beautiful Saturday morning and she was excited about all of the prospects that the day would bring.

She decided to start things out with a cup of one of her favorite teas, which was her own personal blend consisting of loose leaf sarsaparilla root, chamomile, ginger and raspberry. It was the one of her many blends that seemed to truly relax her and give her a sense of wholeness.

As Aset prepared her tea she thought about what she wanted to do for the day. Having been so emotionally detached from everything she really wasn't feeling moved to visit anyone in particular. She thought about stopping by Tisha's house as she hadn't been over there in ages. Tisha was always up and down the highway running her children around from one activity to the next and so she was rarely at home long enough to entertain Aset's company. So she pondered it momentarily but then decided against it. She really wasn't up for a rushed visit.

Instead, Aset wanted to do something that more or less involved only herself. She pulled out her computer to see if there were any good art shows featuring anyone she liked. To her surprise there was! It was set to be held at the ConnerSmith Gallery that afternoon. It was the first day of the Hank Willis Thomas exhibit and she had been dying to see his work in person.

Satisfied with how the day was already shaping up to be Aset finished her tea then went to get dressed. She put on some jeans and a white off the shoulder knit top. However, as she was about to pick out a pair of shoes something began to sort of come alive within her. It was a familiar something. The darkness that had freed itself from her previously was making it's presence known again.

Feeling light-headed Aset plopped down on her bed. Staring straight ahead in a daze she was overcome by such darkness that it as if a dark snake was slithering out of her. Yet at the same time it felt as though it was her slithering out of herself. She began to feel the same magnetic attraction to herself that she had that day in the mirror and it was intoxicating.

Then she looked up and saw what appeared to be a black hole. It wasn't a sinister blackness. In fact, it was hauntingly inviting so much so that Aset gave in to it and allowed it to fully consume her.

Doing so was the most liberating thing that Aset had any recollection of ever doing before. It felt like she had finally freed herself from a prison. She looked around and the darkness seemed to encase her in a warm, homelike feeling. She adjusted herself having remembered how to.

Within seconds she simultaneously had full awareness of her dark form as well as her human form and was fully able to transmutate between both at will. However, now she was more adept at controlling her emotions in her human form. So she didn't have to just be emotionless in order to maintain control over her mind.

In her dark form Aset experienced an expanded version of herself that knew no bounds. She was infinite and illimitable. She was fully able to consume all that was and she did.

For a brief period she transformed as both versions of herself and was amazed at how skillful she was at maintaining her composure. It was a different feeling of power in that despite the limitations of her physical form she had the comfort of knowing that her physical encasement was merely a shell. It was in no way who she was.

The most liberating aspect of what had happened to Aset was that somehow she had broken free from the prison that she had for so long existed in. When she did she remembered who she was and that seemingly opened the door to her transformation back into the fullness of all that she was.

Even in her human form Aset was suddenly in a space where she could easily and willfully transcend all of what previously had been her human weaknesses. So she was beyond the influence of her human feelings, thoughts and emotions. What were once huge, life altering matters were instantly made nonexistent. Debilitating beliefs disappeared. Diseased thoughtforms dissipated all throughout her mind. All that remained were those things that had been true to her form from the start and those things were her desires.

Instantly she felt compelled to realize each one of them. She then began to feel a surge of strong impulses to take various actions toward the ends of doing just that.

So she wanted to paint. She wanted to meet new people and make new connections. She wanted to explore new things. She wanted to try new foods. She wanted to do all of the things that she hadn't before done, but always wanted to do. For the first time in her life all that mattered was that she fully enjoy her life experience.

In that moment Aset had internalized a sunny disposition that somehow breathed new life into her transformed being. Life took on new meaning and was so much more than she remembered. The mastery that she developed over her emotions was eloquent.

Aset felt like a writer, or better yet she felt more like the painter that she was and was anxious to paint her new reality. She got the strongest sensation that life as she knew it was about to take on an entirely new meaning.

She was then able to see the beauty of all that had transpired with her from Amaz's kidnapping of her to the loss of all her material gains and successes. It had all inspired her expansion. It had all inspired her to exist more purposefully and from that moment forward she did.

25

Inspired by the myriad of thoughts racing through her mind regarding all that had transpired Aset found herself sitting in her livingroom painting. She had no recollection of even going to the livingroom let alone getting her paint supplies out and had seemingly, as if by possession, done so.

She concentrated on the various shades and textures of black. Fusing together a variety of colors along with a diverse range of painting techniques Aset's painting was somehow all encompassing. It was a painting that integrated every aspect of the craft onto one canvas.

Aset was impressed. It was like nothing she had ever painted before. It was versatile, innovative and captivating all in one. Aset could barely believe that such a creation had been birthed from her. She must have painted nonstop for hours not feeling the least bit fatigued. Surprisingly she hadn't even needed a break to tend to any physical needs. Moreover, she hadn't noticed that Siris had returned. In that moment she felt superhuman.

Then even more surprisingly looking at the canvas before her Aset was convinced that she was superhuman. Looking intensely at the painting Aset could not believe her eyes.

She had painted a depiction of what she had just experienced. From the looks of it she wasn't necessarily possessed, but she had definitely leaned toward having undergone an out of body experience.

On the canvas was a huge black vortex using painting techniques that were virtually humanly impossible. Besides that it was painted in a way that was absolutely hypnotising, almost as if the painting was bewitched to literally draw the viewer into the painting.

Even Winter seemed to take a liking to it. Winter responded to the painting even more than she did to the obvious differences in Aset.

Inside of the vortex was just as Aset had experienced and it had all that she had ever desired. However, oddly when another viewer looked into the vortex they would somehow *feel* their own desires. It was an experience that was quite unique to the individual viewer.

Aset's desire to be a world renowned artist was felt stronger than any of the others. Secondly was her desire to travel extensively and third was her desire for financial abundance. Most profound was how her desire for a mutually loving, monogamous relationship and was felt, but not as strong as the others. It was still very important to Aset, but in the face of her other desires it wasn't as important as she once thought it was. It was as if the vortex was a well of one's true realized wishes.

As Aset looked at the painting she knew that it was in fact her most impressive work to date. In fact, she felt that it was the one that was going to totally transform her life for the better.

Emanating from the painting itself was a gravitational pull that made it near impossible to turn away as it drew one in further and further. Yet, on face value the painting was nothing spectacular. It simply looked like a canvas that was painted black. However, when gazed upon for more than a couple of seconds the painting instantly drew one in and somehow attracted onlookers to it by what seemed to be some means of an unseen force. Then once paralyzed by its gaze the onlooker was powerless against the vortex.

Smiling at her most recent masterpiece Aset could not wait to unveil it. She sat gleaming from ear to ear as she imagined millions coming in droves to see it.

Then, yanked out of her thoughts, Aset quickly covered it when she heard Siris coming in the door. She was not yet ready for anyone to see it yet, not even Siris.

Aset planned for the unveiling of her painting, which she during that moment officially titled, "The Vortex" to be the most grand of unveilings that she'd ever before had. For the rest of the day Aset could think of nothing else.   She couldn't wait to start reaching out to her most influential and well-connected gallery contacts.

Aset's mind was spinning a thousand miles per second and as a result Siris was virtually invisible to her.   Though it seemed to bother Siris that Aset seemed not to care that he was there Aset was so elated about the prospect of unveiling her painting that she neither felt the slightest bit of guilt nor felt the urge to pretend to.   All that she *did* feel was an overwhelming impulse to get her painting into a gallery by any means possible.   She could think of nothing else, least of all Siris.

So while Siris moped around the living room looking like a lost puppy Aset raced around the apartment like someone bipolar having a manic episode gathering all the business cards and papers with the names, numbers and email addresses of her biggest gallery contacts. She was moving so fast that he could barely figure how to slow her down long enough to say anything to her.

Aset was on a mission to do something huge and Siris was just not a part of that and for that reason he began to fade. The new, expanded version of Aset simply did not invest the time or mental space on matters like Siris or any other mundane affairs nor did it concern her how they responded to her change in disposition. Before, she would obsess over such things, but the newly expanded Aset could care less.

Though hugely connected to Aset's experience was her twin, Bast. As was the usual Bast called Aset after sensing something huge happening.

"Sis what's going on?" Bast inquired excitedly on the other end of the phone.

"B you will never guess. I just painted an absolute masterpiece!" Aset beamed.

"Actually I can. Girl I just saw it in a vision. It's going to be famous all over the world. I saw it! Wow this is so exciting! I can't wait to see it in person!" Bast exclaimed.

"What? You saw the painting in a vision! Now that's creepy," Aset replied.

"Yeah a few hours ago I was having the strangest experience. It was like the whole world opened up to me. It's hard to really even put into words," Bast attempted to explain.

"I know. I know. Trust me you don't have to try. Words could never explain this anyway. I had the same experience. In fact, it's what inspired this painting. It was like something else took over and I couldn't think of anything else except this painting. I'm calling it "The Vortex," Aset said excitedly.

"Oooooooohhhh that's the perfect name for it. Sis I am so happy for you. This is going to be huge. I wish that I was there," Bast squealed.

"Trust me you are here. It feels like it. I felt you with me when I was painting so you must have been here in spirit, literally," Aset chuckled.

"Well I'm going to have to make my way over that way and in the very near future. We need to see each other. This distance is torture. I don't know why I thought this could work. This separation sucks!" Bast fussed.

"We agree. Well I can't wait till you get here. Give me a holler when you get your plane ticket. I can't wait!" Aset exclaimed.

"Will do! Gotta go for now. I'm so proud of you sis. You are amazing and I love you sooooo much. Kiss kiss!" Bast said.

"I love you too and kisses for you too B," Aset said before ending the call.

Aset was beaming after talking to Bast. She always felt that way after she reconnected with her sister. Except this time she was beaming times 100. If there was anyone who related to her experience it was her sister. Their connection was uncanny.

26

Aset was more focused than ever and true to her mission, within just a couple of days she had already gotten a buzz going about "The Vortex." Aset hired an agent to help get the word out having easily convinced him that it was well worth his while and by the time he allowed all of his gallery connections see it the art world was buzzing. It was less than a week later that she got *the* call from a huge gallery contact and it was an opportunity of a lifetime.

"Hello may I speak to Aset Bridges?" a voice on the other end of the phone asked.

"Yes, this is she," Aset answered with a hint of curiosity in her voice.

"Hi Ms. Bridges! This is Carrie Stone from the Angoran Gallery. I recently saw your piece entitled "The Vortex" and let me first say that I was absolutely mesmerized by it. I mean I am just blown away by your artistry," the caller gleamed.

Typically gallery owners would contact the agent of the artist, however this call was an exception to the rule. Carrie Stone needed no introductions as her art gallery, Angoran was quite well-known all throughout the art community. As well, Carrie Stone as it's owner was quite renowned. Aset was near star struck as she struggled to respond.

"Oh thank you so much Ms. Stone," Aset replied bashfully, "that is quite the compliment coming from you."

"I was calling to ask if you would do us the honor of allowing Angoran to be the gallery to unveil and officially introduce your masterpiece to the world. It would truly be our honor," Carrie inquired.

Aset was expecting to hear from her agent telling her that several galleries were interested, but she had no idea she'd hear directly from such an esteemed gallery and so quickly. She didn't even need to ponder it.

She knew exactly what she was going to do. So without hesitation she responded.

"It would be my pleasure Ms. Stone. Your gallery would be the perfect venue to unveil "The Vortex," Aset responded excitedly.

Aset couldn't believe it! She'd gotten a call back from the Angoran Gallery in New York City! It was one of New York's top modern art museums and Aset was so honored to be a featured artist there.

Carrie had seen "The Vortex" at a viewing along with a colleague and after witnessing it was anxious to be the first to host the unveiling so she didn't hesitate for a moment before contacting Aset. For so long Aset dreamt of seeing her artwork on the walls of such a prestigious gallery and she was overjoyed at the prospect of such a dream coming true. It seemed that her vortex was very real and her desires were quickly becoming her reality.

"Wow! Well that's fantastic Ms. Bridges. I am so honored. We'd like to roll out the showing in the very near future so I will have my planners get on it right away. I'd like to schedule it within the next few weeks so if your agent can give me a date that works best for you I can get right on it," Carrie replied.

"Absolutely, we'll look at my calendar and get back to you within the next couple of days. Thank you so much for this wonderful invitation and I look forward to this venture," Aset answered.

"I do as well. This is as much an honor to us. I for one am very anxious to see the art world's response to your profound work. So I look forward to hearing back from you within the next couple of days Ms. Bridges and again it is truly my honor to host this showing for you," Carrie said graciously.

"Thank you Ms. Stone and you be well," Aset concluded.

Aset ended the call buzzing with anticipation. She felt so high that she thought at any moment she would take off in flight. It was like the painting had awakened her from the dead.

The showing of "The Vortex" was sure to be her biggest showing yet and there was nothing that could dare take the joy of that away from her. Since the other side of Aset had awakened she was able to experience emotions at a much heightened level than before. More than that she had command over them such that those that she wanted to experience in a heightened state, such as joy, she could. Meanwhile, those that she wanted to minimize she could and it was with the quickness and slightest of thought.

Her thoughtforms were no longer lightning spears that attacked her. Instead, her thoughtforms were whatever she commanded them to be and that changed the entire course of how Aset existed in her human form.

Thoughtforms were the architects of her human reality. In fact, she had realized that unbeknownst to most every person's thoughtforms created their individual reality. Collectively, their thoughtforms created their collective, common experience. So Aset's new ability to control her thoughts at will was a major advancement, not only for her, but for any others who also realized their power to do the same.

The more Aset gazed at "The Vortex" the more empowered she became. It had become her infinite source of power. She began to feel invincible. For Aset there was nothing and noone who could ever again force her back into the mental prison that she had so long existed in.

She couldn't believe the freedom that she had so long deprived herself of. She still was not sure how she managed to break free of it and she didn't much care. What was most important to Aset was her freedom of limitations. No job, no government, no man, no religion, no beliefs, not even her own thoughts would ever again imprison Aset. Of that she was certain and it was a certainty that was just as much determined as it was divinely willful. Aset had transformed into a higher consciousness that was beyond the influence of anything human.

Over the course of the next several days Aset spent the bulk of her time playing around a bit with those powers. Day in and day out as life happened Aset used it as an opportunity to test her new abilities. Each time without fail she reigned supreme. The more successful she was the more comfortable she became with embracing her new self. She also became that much more joyful about life.

Siris and others could not understand what was happening to Aset. In many cases, particularly that of Siris, Aset was tested in the manner of provocation. Siris must have pulled every stunt that he could conjure to bring Aset down from the incessant high that she was on. He couldn't understand why she was always so damn happy nor did he have the ability to share in it so in his frustration he tried to destroy it.

For Aset, it was as if her state of interminable happiness was her force field and nothing could penetrate it. Besides that the more momentum her happiness gained the more doors began to open for her, the more opportunities opened up for her, the more favorable things were for her and the more inspired she became to pursue more.

For Aset there was no end to what she could accomplish or what she was able to realize. She was empowered to have all that she ever desired and so she went after just that.

Meanwhile, the more people and circumstances attempted to obstruct her path the more powerful she became. It seemed that with each attempt she learned something more about herself and was better able to hone her skills.

Aset could feel that it was only a matter of time before she would be completely free, even from her human form if she so desired. She was beginning to feel that not even Amaz could hold her back any longer.

27

The closer the date of the showing got the more more anxious Aset became. It was all that Aset could think of. As she waited Aset experienced a burst of creative inspiration. She must have completed at least 5 additional pieces, each more mystifying than the last.

"The Vortex" turned out to be the origination of a much bigger story as Aset's additional paintings went on to tell a much deeper story. It was a story that Aset wasn't even sure the world was ready for. So she decided to keep a lid on the rest of the collection until she felt the time was right.

What it revealed was seemingly more than the human mind was currently able to conceptualize. It simply defied description.

More than that as a collection all of the paintings together in the same physical space seemed to have an irresistible alluring force that many probably would not even be able to handle. It was an all consuming force of power analogous to that of a black hole.

Essentially it was Aset in all of her natural glory. If words could describe it almost felt like it sucked the viewer into a sort of alternate reality that, like "The Vortex." was unique to the viewer.

Each reality seemed to be based on the true desires of the individual viewer that was largely based on the strongest of their desires most activated within the person at the time of the viewing.

For Aset, it transported her to a reality where everyone seemed to have a heightened awareness of their interconnectedness to one another. Yet, at the same time they seemed to be very much aware of their own individual passions and were quite focused on them. Because of this they were very drawn to those much like themselves, which made for a very harmonious world. It was like Aset's nirvana and was quickly becoming her newest addiction as she began to spend more and more time with her paintings so that she could remain in her alternate reality as much as possible.

In some ways Aset thought that others should experience her collection. On the other hand, she didn't believe that most were ready for such a revelation. She knew that the paintings could potentially have a devastating effect on someone who wasn't quite evolved and in-tuned enough with the more spiritually evolved aspect of themself. Thus, she decided against sharing the entire collection and decided to for the time being only reveal the single original piece of "The Vortex."

It seemed that once the word had gotten out about the surreal painting the more people became obsessed with an insatiable urge to witness it for themselves. It was anticipated that people from all over the country were planning to attend the initial showing. Since then, the Angoran Gallery had to require tickets be purchased with appointed times assigned to each in order to accommodate all of those who wanted to see the painting.

Aset was beginning to question whether she was going to attend the showing as she didn't really want so much attention. She enjoyed her privacy and wasn't sure if she was ready to give that up. So she was still undecided as to what she was going to do.

As a result, Carrie Stone's PR team was up in arms about Aset's hesitation about attending the showing. They had already formulated an entire PR campaign that more or less required her attendance. They hadn't pitched her as the sequestered type. When they met with her they saw her as outgoing, sociable and attractive with all the other makings of a PR goldmine. Nonetheless, Aset was adamant about needing time to consider what she felt most comfortable with.

Aset's local associates and colleagues had already begun ringing her phone like crazy all buzzing about the showing as well, all suddenly asking to hook up and all acting as if Aset was some mega superstar.

It seemed they were even more excited than she was about the showing. They had all planned to attend and the closer they got to the date of the showing the more anxious everyone got.

With all the buzz about Aset's painting she wondered if the painting was bewitched. Everyone's obsession with it seemed somehow aberrant. Often when she engaged in general conversation the topic of the painting would always seemingly sneak in and take over and dominate the conversation like a super force. It was like the painting itself was a higher intelligence.

Eventually, the painting became the voice that Aset had recently lost that day in the tub. It became the glue that reconnected her mind to her body. It became all that manifested her into human, physical form. It became the explanation for life as she had come to understand and know it.

What Aset would soon learn was that "The Vortex" would become the door to her new beginning. Without yet clearly understanding she felt this. It was the one thing that comforted her in the midst of her life issues, which still launched occasional attacks. It was what made life with the likes of Siris and his drama bearable. In a world of confusion and disorder "The Vortex" made sense of things, which was part of its allure.

By the day of the showing the unveiling of "The Vortex" seemed like a national holiday. People from all over the country had come to witness it. There were at least 5,000 in attendance over the course of the entire day. Though to the disappointment of many Aset decided not to attend, at least not openly. She actually was there lingering in the wings accompanied by her twin sister, Bast and Siris dressed in jeans, a black leather jacket and a large, floppy though very stylish black felt wide brimmed hat, which somewhat disguised her identity to those who may have otherwise recognized her.

As she watched several people experience "The Vortex" she was always left aghast at how personally it impacted each person. Yet one aspect of the experience that everyone seemed to have in common was that "The Vortex" somehow spoke to them. It was always very difficult for people to articulate exactly how, but "The Vortex" had a way of communicating to the viewer by way of thought. It sort of gave them a feeling about the veracity of the thought by way of an indescribable sensation. So from a series of feelings one knew exactly what "The Vortex" was communicating. It was quite uncanny.

After finally experiencing "The Vortex" for herself Bast was the most proud and impressed with her sister. She was truly her number one fan.

As they both stood in the gallery staring at the painting with huge smiles plastered across their faces Bast said with more pride than the universe could probably handle, "Sis words cannot express just how very, very proud of you I am. You are absolutely amazing and you are so deserving of all the success that you are receiving right now. I wish a super huge amount of abundant success that causes you to soar far beyond your imagination. You are truly a masterpiece, a work of art sis and I love you!"

Aset was so choked up by all of the beautiful things that her sister had just said that she had to struggle to form words as the tears rolled down her face. Moreover, coming from her sister made it the greatest honor of all.

Struggling to hold it together Aset replied, "B I could have never done this without your constant support. You are such a huge part of the inspiration to my art."

Then bursting into a stream of unstoppable tears Aset hugged Bast tightly until they work both sobbing like they did when they used to watch chick flicks together. The remainder of the evening was absolutely magical for Aset and she hated to see it end.

The next morning Siris returned to D.C., which gave Bast and Aset the time they needed to catch up and enjoy some much needed time together. They acted like two high strung teenagers partying and enjoying New York City to the fullest. They enjoyed all of their favorite cuisines from Thai to Soul Food they must have sampled a restaurant in very burrough. They went to the movies, caught a show and Bast even took Aset shopping. They celebrated in every way possible and by the time the weekend was over they were both exhausted. They were at the same time really sad to have to say goodbye to one another as they both had to return to their lives.

They both made a vow to one another to come back together again as the separation was killing them. They didn't know how, but they somehow knew within the depths of them that soon they would be together again and so they parted ways both trusting in the strength of that mutual desire.

Then over the next several months people continued to come to the Angoran Gallery in droves to see "The Vortex" all reporting similar profound experiences. As a result Aset's entire life changed. Her name became one of the biggest in art. Hers was said to be the most insightful masterfully crafted pieces of art to ever grace the planet.

28

Meanwhile, as Aset's popularity grew Siris seemed all the more resentful of her. He wasn't quite able to deal with her success and all of the attention it garnered.

It had been close to 5 months since Aset and Siris had in Siris' mind 'made up.' For him despite her change in emotional disposition they had been doing quite well for the most part. He was doing backflips trying to win Aset's trust back and the part of her that still seemed human was able to convince him that he had. However, the other part of her that was more preoccupied with much bigger things, like her expanded Self and her newest creative masterpiece, could have cared less.

Si just didn't hold the same position of importance in Aset's life since she had come to the realization that there were way more important things to focus on. The only thing that seemed to matter to Aset was finding a way to return to what she began to view as her dark nirvana.

She knew that in order to do that she would have to once and for all get more control over her mind and thereby subdue the lightning spears that were still occasionally launching attacks against her. The momentary bouts of dominance over the lightning spears was more power than Aset had ever experienced and thus she developed a craving for it. So she wanted more and somehow Siris was the key to that! For that reason and that reason alone she kept him around.

Given that, a lot had changed between them in Aset's new sense of being. She began to enjoy the fact that Siris' comings and goings no longer phased her. After all it wasn't so long ago that she would obsess over such nonsensical things.

She also enjoyed how life's day-to-day concerns no longer consumed her. What once were seemingly monumental life matters, like Siris' cheating, had then become irrelevant details that she no longer *worried* about. By way of all of the challenges that Siris had posed, Aset was becoming more and more empowered and in the process her dominance was quickly gaining momentum. As a result, Aset was gradually creating a reality where she did whatever she wanted to do whenever she wanted to do it and it was so liberating.

Her newfound freedom was a constant reminder that she never wanted to be confined by the limitations of her mind again. For so long Aset had limited herself to the expectations and desires of everyone but herself. She had limited herself to rehearsed responses to things. She limited herself to accept undesirable circumstances and conditions that others put on her. So finally coming to the realization that she didn't have to succumb to any of that was liberating and the most clear indication of that was soon to be revealed.

Though Aset was back in the rhythm of her dealings with Siris where she spent the bulk of her time with him she remained emotionally detached as doing so was the best way to respond to his increasingly jaundiced attitude towards her. It turned out that having such a disposition would serve her well because Siris decided to pull his biggest stunt yet.

Since their reunion Aset quickly learned not to give her attention to all of Siris' newfound antics. Apparently he thought that since Aset had taken him back that by default made him quite the ladies man. So his phone rang a lot more often and he'd run outside to take the calls. He'd also taken to texting a lot and was therefore receiving text messages at all hours of the night. More than that his ego had become so big that Aset doubted the universe was big enough to house it.

She wasn't sure if with his latest stunt he was trying to get a rise out of her or if he was trying to test her intelligence or perhaps he just stopped caring about the relationship all together and was just going through the motions by staying in it. One couldn't say what Siris' motivation was for doing what he did. At any rate in the weirdest kind of way it ended up being just the push that Aset needed to fully come into the fullness of her power and finally bring an end to the remnants of the war that was still active within her, even if just minimally.

One weekend Siris had told Aset that they would not link up until Sunday because he had a wedding to attend. So throughout the course of the weekend he called her sparingly, but not nearly as much as usual. Even more out of character was that on both Friday and Saturday he called her to say goodnight a lot earlier than usual. Though, none of that phased her any as she had become increasingly more fond of and happily welcomed time to herself.

Then, as planned for that Sunday she and Siris linked up. Siris asked Aset to come over to his place and so she did. Seemingly *comfortable* again Siris was back to being the arrogant jerk that he always had been snapping at Aset for minor things trying to make molehills into mountains. However, it was no surprise to Aset so she did not let it bother her.

So once Aset settled in she noticed that there were some women's personal hygiene products in the bathroom that were not hers. Being in the space that she was about things Aset didn't feel moved to say anything about it so she continued on as if oblivious to it.

However, Siris' messiness didn't stop there. When they went to bed Aset smelled a woman's perfume on her pillowcase. The scent was so strong that it was as if the woman had sprayed it on the pillowcase purposely. Still Aset said nothing.

Aset was very pleased with the progress she'd made. She knew that the old Aset would have gone off on Siris, but the new Aset had absolutely no desire to control Siris or do backflips to get him to change for her. In the bliss of her new found freed mental space she had come to realize that her joy in life was never about controlling Siris or anyone else, but instead it was about controlling how she felt about herself. So in that moment she cared too much about herself to be concerned about Siris and his antics and so she wasn't.

Aset had discovered her true desires had nothing to do with Siris and everything to do with herself. She was on a journey to discovering her own bliss within herself and it was in that moment that she realized that she and she alone was finally fully in control of her reality. She realized that it always was her.

So for the first time it no longer depended on Siris having to do right by her. It no longer had to with Siris wanting to be with her and her having to be a certain way or do certain things in an attempt to manipulate him into doing so. Her happiness was no longer contingent on the hopes that she could somehow keep Siris' focus on her long enough to make him not desire any other woman but her.

In that moment Aset realized that it was in fact all of the contrast and negativity that Siris had brought to her life that was the catalyst for her very timely enlightenment. It was no longer about his lying, cheating, belittling or blaming. It wasn't about his demonization of women. It wasn't about his disregard for all that she was. She was in that moment most beautiful. She was so beautiful and it was all about her very iridescent beauty that then bright enough for the entire world to see. It was all about Aset and Aset alone. Siris and no one else mattered. Finally she realized that the only one that bought Aset happiness was Aset.

So she had not a thought about who Siris had spent the weekend with or why he would be so careless as to not clear out the evidence. She only thought of herself and what she wanted and it was the most heavenly realization.

So while she was deep in thought she gazed down at Siris. It all felt very much like a dream as she looked at him. Suddenly it was as if he was a stranger, an actual stranger! She had no idea *who* was lying next to her.

In her dreamlike state Aset looked at Siris' face and she simply didn't recognize him. She grabbed his hand and they had absolutely no familiarity. She inhaled deeply to try to catch his scent, but it was so faint that it was barely perceptible. Eventually, as she tried to discern his overall person she realized that he was indiscernible.

Then as if sensing her gaze Siris woke up reminding Aset that it wasn't at all a dream. With a serene look on her face Aset smiled at him lovingly as if he was the love of her life and the man that she had always dreamed of. Almost blushing Siris smiled back at Aset surprised to be awakened in such a way.

Breaking the silence Aset spoke softly saying, "I dreamt of something so wonderful last night my love."

"Oh yeah, well it must have been about me because you certainly are glowing this morning," Siris said with an arrogant grin taking great pride in his work.

"Hmmm perhaps, but not directly. I dreamt that I was living the life of my dreams," Aset gleamed as if she actually was.

"Wow, well that must have been some dream." Siris said dismissively.

Having made some decisions while she lie awake deep in thought Aset responded saying, "So as I slept I dreamt of the most blissful life where I had finally manifested all that I had ever desired."

Pausing while basking in the moment of it all she continued, "I was in a most lovingly blissful relationship with a man who wanted the same things in life that I wanted. There were no conflicts because we were such a match. There was only unconditional love. There was no pressure to be anything but who we both wanted to be. There was only unconditional love. There was no dishonesty. The best part was that there was simply an honest commitment to continue to grown into the best of who we both were in our own truths, which made it the most beautiful commitment ever," Aset said smiling.

Feeling anger beginning to surge Siris begrudgingly replied, "So what is all of that supposed to mean? You feel like we don't have any of that?"

"No I don't. I see the obvious in that we want very different lives. You want a one-sided open relationship and I want a mutually exclusive relationship with a man that wants the same and who is committed only to the betterment of himself as am I," Aset calmly replied.

"Aset what is this about? Is there something that you want to say to me?" Siris asked getting more annoyed with each word.

"Since you ask, which means you're open to hear me I do. Do you or do you not desire to be in the same type of relationship that I just described to you?" Aset asked blankly.

Siris took a long pause before responding and when he did he was visibly exasperated.

"Look Aset I see what you're getting at and I told you before that I don't see anything wrong with men having more than one woman. It's been going on since the beginning of time and it's not gonna stop now. As far as I'm concerned that's something the women need to work out among one another. With that I'm done with it because I'm not getting into another long drawn out debate about this with you," Siris said with finality.

Siris was tired of debating with Aset about the subject of men having more than one woman. In fact, he was tired of feeling like he had to answer to her about what he was doing. As far as he was concerned he gave Aset the world. He treated her like a queen. He spent more time with her than any of the other women got and he spoiled her rotten. He felt like he at least had the decency to not overtly cheat on her. In fact, he went out of his way to be discreet and for that reason he felt like Aset didn't appreciate what a good thing she had in a man like him. Besides that he really loved her. If he didn't care he wouldn't bother trying to prevent her from finding out about the other women. So he was taken aback by Aset's response.

For several moments Aset sat in silence. She inhaled and exhaled slowly and deeply, closed her eyes and momentarily retreated back into her thoughts. Then struck by a strong and unreflective urge to act she spoke.

"Hmmm, well I'm not going to be able to do that," Aset said calmly.

Then suddenly overcome by an even more intense feeling of inner peace and having a strong impulse to leave Aset decided to do just that. So while Siris sat on the bed Aset promptly and quietly gathered her belongings, sat Siris' apartment key on the nightstand and left without saying another word.

Siris was in shock. He wasn't quite sure how to take this Aset. He'd never seen this side of her before and didn't quite know how to respond. There was such a finality in her exit that he knew that it was real.

He knew that this time no matter what he said or did Aset was not coming back. He knew that she meant exactly what she said, but for the life of him he couldn't figure out where it all came from all of a sudden.

Still absorbing the shock of what had so abruptly transpired Siris sat frozen on the bed. It seemed that all in a matter of seconds Aset had spoken her peace, grabbed her belongings and made her exit.

Besides the abruptness of what had happened Siris was also quite taken aback at how calm Aset was. She had the most uncanny sense of inner peace. Perhaps it was the witnessing of that which caused Siris to sort of freeze up and not attempt to stop her like he usually did. Perhaps he knew deep down inside that Aset truly did deserve more than he was willing to give her. So with that Siris sat frozen in his own pain and fear of facing life without Aset.

Meanwhile, Aset made her way out of the building having finally realized that though misery needs company happiness walks alone. With that she was overcome with the most intense feeling of happiness that she had ever felt.

29

After leaving, feeling not even the least bit regretful Aset was suddenly struck with the keenest sense of knowing that all that she desired was about to come to fruition. She could feel it through and through. Leaving Siris didn't feel like a loss, it felt like a very much anticipated beginning of something beautiful.

She had finally found her voice. She had finally realized her truth and it didn't matter to her how anyone but her felt about it. It only mattered how she felt and that she felt good about what she had just done.

Suddenly a rush of feeling came over Aset. She could feel again. The very depths of her emotions could be felt once again. She was no longer the emotionless shell of a person that she had become, particularly with Siris. Not only could she feel, but she was in total control of *how* she felt.

Aset felt like an alchemist. She felt that at her command she could transform any emotion into one that she wanted. In doing so, she finally realized herself as the Dark Goddess and as she did the powers within her awakened.

The next week, wanting to again experience the happiness that she enjoyed the last time she saw Bast, Aset was compelled to drive to the Angoran gallery in New York. So she got dressed, got in the car and got on the road. Once she arrived it was crowded as had been the case for the past several months so she had to make her way through a bit of a crowd just to get somewhat close to her painting. As she stood gazing at "The Vortex" she began to feel spacey. She wondered if she had ventured into a dream state, but she was wide awake. She wondered if it was that her mind had again distanced her so much from her physical reality that she could no longer recognize where she was with her physical senses. Yet, when she looked around the gallery everything was as it should be or at least she thought it was.

Her eyes were suddenly drawn to what was the most handsome and intriguing man that she had ever laid eyes on. Strangely he seemed very familiar. He stared back at her as if the feeling was mutual.

For both of them it seemed like they had always known one another and unbeknownst to them they had. They were always the divine match waiting to happen. The truth was that they had always been in close proximity to one another. They had always shared one another's desires. They had always harnessed a love for one another. It was all waiting for them in "The Vortex."

Just then Aset noticed that *everything* around her had changed. She saw things that she had often thought of having and hoped that she would someday obtain appear right before her very eyes. Aset blinked a few times to make sure that she was not dreaming. She looked around and saw the home of her dreams and it had in it everything that she'd ever dreamed of.

She sat looking around in wonderment of her own creation. Then touching the plushness of the comforter atop the queen-sized bed that she sat upon in awe of her manifestation Aset smiled and let herself fall back on the bed staring up at the high ceilings of her luxurious master suite.

She thought to herself, "I did it! I finally did it! How much better can this get?"

Aset then smiled soaking in the awesomeness of the manifestation before her. All around her was the most luxurious furnishings she had ever seen up close and personal. Her room was like something out of a magazine.

Just as she'd always wanted her room furnishings were all off white with accents of lavender. She had a plush custom-made round bed covered with the softest mixture of silk and textured fabrics. The bedding was so soft that she thought she might melt in it.

Just below the bed was a thick, lavish off white rug that gave one the sensation of walking on air. Then, to her surprise, as she looked down barely noticeable as she blended in was Winter sprawled out on the rug as if it were her personal bed. Aset smiled to herself comforted to see a familiar face as it confirmed the realness of the experience. Winter looked just as pleased with the new abode as was Aset.

On the wall behind her was the most elaborate piece of artistry she'd ever seen. It was a hand scorned iron screed that looked something like a lotus. On each side of her bed were 2 burl wood inlaid nightstands and on the other side of the room adjacent to her bed was a matching chest of drawers. To the left of Aset was an exquisite velvet covered chaise lounge facing a stone fireplace accompanied by Aset's own artwork on the wall above in what appeared to be a reading area.

Looking around the room Aset thought that surely she was in heaven. She realized that she had finally created it for herself by way of her own mind and it was the most exhilarating sense of power that she had ever experienced.

Anxious to see the rest of her phenomenal manifestation like a kid visiting Disney World for the first time Aset jumped up running through what was soon to be discovered was her very own castle. The rest of her house was even more extravagantly decorated than her room.

There were 3 great rooms, 8 bathrooms, 6 bedroom suites, a restaurant sized chef-style kitchen, a basement that was the full length size of the house and a 4-car garage. Most astounding was that the entire house was decorated with Aset's own artwork! She was in awe of herself and was taken aback by the ingenuity of her own work.

As she basked in the bliss of her own creation she kept wondering how much better it could all get. Just as that thought crossed her mind Aset had a strong sense that the best was yet to come and she would soon learn that she couldn't have been more right.

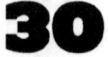

Embracing her from behind, entrancing her with his touch was the culmination of all of Aset's well-deserved blessings. In human form he was the story of her evolution. From the Dark Goddess to the disregarded, witless bitch to the sagacious intelligence he had magnetically maintained his gravitational link to her, inseparable, indivisible and indestructible.

Unable to suppress her curiosity Aset spun around to see him. He was the man from the gallery and he was exactly as she'd felt him.

Being a visual artist did not lend itself to Aset's ability to visualize her ideal man, so she had to feel him. By way of feelings she could describe every detail of her ideal guy and then right before her he stood. He was even better than she remembered. He was the guy from the Angoran gallery in New York and he was the man of her dreams.

Part of her couldn't believe it and part of her expected it. She felt it when she met him, but wasn't yet ready to *see* him and so she didn't until the day at the gallery.

The fact was they'd crossed paths many times before. They'd been on the train together. They'd seen one another at the bookstore. They'd even seen one another at an art showing or two as they both shared a love for the craft. They'd been in the same grocery store before and once they even said hello to one another. Though, despite all of their chance encounters the time was not yet right for them to officially meet and so they didn't.

Yet in that moment there she stood seeing him and feeling him in all of his glory and it was the most wonderful experience. She'd always felt him around in the recesses of her mind even during the worst of her relationships. Even most recently with Siris she knew that the man of her true desires was always very near and silently she maintained her determination to manifest him into her life.

Momentarily recalling everything that she had gone through in one failed relationship after another, heartbreak after heartbreak, outrage after outrage caused a tear to roll down Aset's cheek. It was a tear that held all of the growing pains of evolution. It held all of the despair and hopelessness that she felt during her time of bondage in his world. It also held the joy of a new day in the anticipated arrival of a resuscitated, reawakened, returned new wombman.

As the single tear fell from her face hitting the floor like a ton of bricks Aset simultaneously said 1000 goodbyes to her hellish reality while looking deeply into the heavenly eyes of her man warmly saying, "Peace, my God."

In them she felt the warmth, love, kindness and peace that she had so long craved and so long coveted. As she stared into them dreamy-eyed Aset suddenly felt a compelling force of singularity and she was again ONE.

In rediscovering her self-created reality Aset went on to live out what others would have considered something that only happens in fairytales. However, it was far from a fairytale. It was very real. Aset had come to know an invaluable realization, which was that she and she alone, not some external force was and had always been the creator of her reality from the largest of experiences down to the most minute of details.

She, like the other Goddesses who had made their way to Earth, were quite powerful in their being. However, after being stripped away from their Source a large part of those powers went dormant and would remain so until they learned to awaken them. The awakening process proved quite difficult for the Goddesses in the face of succumbing to their humanness and so they remained imprisoned by their own minds. It took the most sadistic of treatment at the hands of the God Amaz in both his true and his human form to rouse the Goddesses to awakening.

Nonetheless, awakened Aset was and there was no turning back. She would never turn back to the miserable reality that she'd once known.

Meanwhile, those who had not experienced "The Vortex" remained trapped by the limitations of their physical existence. They remained as prisoners to a dictatorship of repressed emotions merely existing as a shadow of themselves. In the perpetual certitude that life was meant to be toilsome they persisted as a lingering ominous cloud of damnation. Among them was Siris and Tisha, who for the rest of their existence would be reminded of who she was whenever they looked up at the dark sky. She was the Dark Goddess, the yoniverse that was the self-created prison of their minds.

For her they were all a forgotten memory of a distant reality as she stood in amazement at what was then her new life. Then as if again reading her mind Aset's phone rang. Before answering she already knew who it was.

"Bast! Are you experiencing this?" Aset answered bursting with excitement.

"Yes sis! If I wasn't living this moment right now I wouldn't believe it and guess what?" Bast replied matching Aset's excitement as there was a ringing of Aset's doorbell.

"No! You're not!" Aset answered running to the door nearly about to run herself over as she couldn't get to the door fast enough.

Aset arrived at the door and gasped before anxiously turning the knob with the phone still to her ear. She then swung the door open to find a smiling Bast with the phone still to her ear as well until they both dropped their phones and embraced one another as if they had been estranged for several lifetimes.

As they embraced one another Aset caught a vision that Bast had also broken free and reinvented her reality and in it she, accompanied by Nigga, lived right next door to her beloved twin sister. For Aset, Bast's presence needed no explanation. Without being told she knew all that had transpired for Bast.

Like Aset, Bast realized her true desires and to her surprise they included and were a match to Nigga's. Once they both came into alignment with who they truly were and what they truly wanted they realized that their souls were meant to grow together and so they did. Nigga continued to come into his Godhood and freely gave Bast the room to evolve into the Goddess that she was. Together they co-created the most blissful new reality.

So there Bast stood, looking at the smile on Aset's face and feeling the love emanate from her heart knowing that her sister had finally harnessed the courage to welcome happiness into her life. For both sisters what happened was more than they had ever imagined and in the beauty of that moment Aset felt gracious. She felt joyous. She felt the euphoria of a thousand heavens. She felt the wholeness of her being. Mostly she felt all that she had finally given birth to as pure blissful satisfaction.

If you enjoyed this book or received value from it in any way, then I'd like to ask you for a favor. Would you be kind enough to leave a review for this book on Amazon? It'd be greatly appreciated!

About the Author....

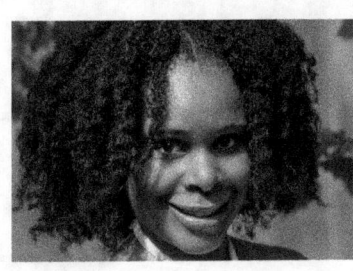

Amirah Bellamy is truly a bonafide artist of many crafts. In addition to being a novelist she's also a Kemetic yoga instructor and singer (check out her cd entitled "Raising Love Consciousness also available on Amazon). Amirah grew up in the DC Metro area, which is where much of the inspiration to many of her novels came from. She developed a fondness for the sci-fi genre as a child watching shows like Star Trek and movies like Star Wars. Eventually, her fascination with the metaphysical evolved into research, which then evolved into novel writing. Today, as a novelist she now welcomes you into her creative universe.

To learn more about Amirah Bellamy

email.... twenty6dimension@gmail.com

or

visit..... www.EthericRealmsInv.com

Black Wombman

**Other books by this author also available
(Visit www.EthericRealmsInv.com to learn
more!) ....**

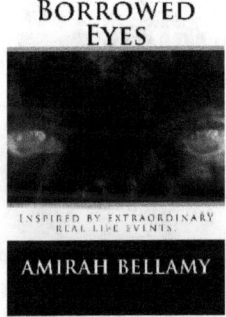

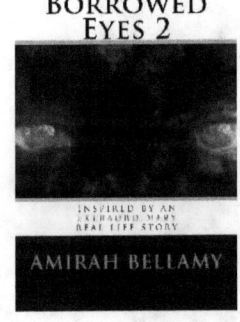

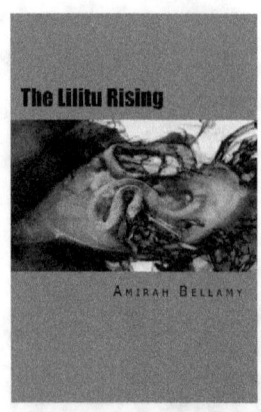

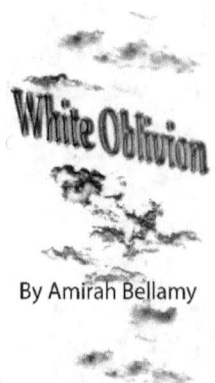

By Amirah Bellamy

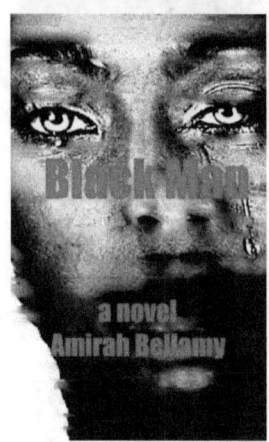

www.ingramcontent.com/pod-product-compliance
Lightning Source LLC
Chambersburg PA
CBHW062126280526
45788CB00001B/72